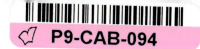
# THE FOOD CURE

## FOR KIDS

# THE FOOD CURE

## FOR KIDS

### A Nutritional Approach to Your Child's Wellness

Natalie Geary, MD
Oz Garcia, PhD

LYONS PRESS
Guilford, Connecticut

*An imprint of Globe Pequot Press*

To buy books in quantity for corporate use
or incentives, call **(800) 962-0973**
or e-mail **premiums@GlobePequot.com**.

Lyons Press is an imprint of Globe Pequot Press.

Text design by Sheryl Kober
Layout by Kirsten Livingston
Project manager: Kristen Mellitt

Library of Congress Cataloging-in-Publication Data is available on file.

ISBN 978-0-7627-5886-9

Printed in the United States of America

10 9 8 7 6 5 4 3 2 1

Neither the publisher nor the authors is engaged in rendering professional advice or services
to the individual reader. Please consult your physician before following any of the suggestions
herein; also consult your physician about any health problems you or your child may be
having. If your child is taking prescription drugs, do not give them any supplements until
you have consulted your health professional.

This book is dedicated to my children, Isabelle, Lily Rose, and Adelaide, who have taught me more about being a parent than any textbook in pediatrics and who were so sweet teaching me; and to my patients and their families, who allowed me the honor of participating in their care.

—*Natalie Geary*

To all parents everywhere who are dedicated to their children's health and happiness, but especially to Mom for raising me to be who I am; to my Dad to whom I am eternally grateful; and to my late beloved Kosmos, who gave me so much joy.

—*Oz Garcia*

# Contents

# Introduction

Parents hear it all the time. Tiny voices, squeaking out from behind those tear-filled puppy dog eyes, calling out, "Mommy, make me feel better." It can be so frustrating for moms (and dads, too) when you know that your child is just not feeling well and you don't know what to do about it. Most of the time, it's not a major illness that's bothering your child; it's a chronic earache, or a tummy that's upset, or an inexplicable something that causes your child to say, "I don't feel so good."

What if we could help you prevent these kinds of complaints before they begin? That's what this book is about. It's about using food—plain old everyday food—to help your child feel better. There are no special diets required. You don't have to be a gourmet chef. You don't have to hide vegetables in birthday cake. You don't have to spend extra money. You don't have to make your kids feel different or excluded because they can't have what all the other kids are having. All you need to do is understand some of the basics of how little bodies work and how the foods they eat influence their physical and mental health. That's what you'll find in the chapters to come.

**What if we could help you prevent these kinds of complaints before they begin? It's about using food—plain old everyday food—to help your child feel better.**

In Part I, you'll learn what makes kids tick. You'll discover how to find out if your child is one of the earache, tummy ache, tired, irritable, I-don't-want-to-go-to-school kinds of kids; how evolution has shaped our biology and how current agricultural practices are wreaking havoc with our digestive systems; how our kids' immune systems work and how they're influenced by what they consume; and why allergies and food sensitivities are so prevalent in our society today.

In Part II, you'll learn about specific foods and food groups, and why so many of them are so good for us—and so bad for us when they're overconsumed. You'll learn why cutting out carbohydrates can be devastating for children's health and why eating too many of the wrong kind of carbs can be just as bad. You'll find out about the pros and cons of wheat, dairy, proteins, and fats. And you'll be introduced to probiotics, the friendly bacteria that form a natural defense barrier against harmful bacteria and toxins, and that we all need for healthy digestive and immune system function.

Part III gets into some of the newest food-related issues that kids are dealing with today. Food has become an incredibly sensitive topic for children, and parents are often at a loss as to how to handle these delicate situations. This section of the book deals with the obesity epidemic that is facing our country today, and how you can help your child deal with the subject of food and the issues that surround it. And finally, the last chapter addresses the fact that food is not the only influence on a child's mental and physical fitness. Any program of good health has to include sleep, exercise, and stress relief.

**The source of many of our young patients' illnesses and behavioral problems was as serious and as simple as a nutritional imbalance.**

Throughout the book you will find stories of patients we have seen over the years. The names have been changed to protect their privacy, but these stories represent typical scenarios we see over and over again in our practices. At the end of each chapter, you will find questions to take to your own pediatrician that will make it easier for you to focus the conversation on issues that we are discussing in each chapter. These questions are simply suggestions of things you might like to ask your doctor yourself. Many of them are questions that parents have asked us over the years. Our hope is that they, along with the quick chapter review of the "take-home" points, will trigger questions of your own about your child's health.

What sets this book apart is that it addresses children's overall well-being—healthy digestive function, cognitive performance, healthy hormone development, a more resilient immune system, increased energy and focus—by integrating traditional pediatric medicine with expert nutrition.

When Oz Garcia and I met at a Fourth-of-July birthday party for a mutual friend, we instantly knew that our philosophies were compatible. What began with a "you two probably have a lot in common" introduction became an evening-long conversation about our mutual concern: the role of nutrition in the health of America's children today. We discussed the ballooning problems of obesity and diabetes in young children and teens, as well as issues of lack of energy in children of all ages and the inability to focus well in class.

Although we were trained very differently, we had come to the same conclusions about the current state of children's health in America: that the source of many of our young patients' illnesses and behavioral problems was as serious and as simple as a nutritional imbalance. We also realized that we shared a common goal: to promote, foster, and teach parents and their children to have a healthy relationship with food and eating—one that is not based on tricks or fads, but is instead practical, realistic, and will last them a lifetime.

I am a classically trained pediatrician who has studied Ayurvedic medicine and practices "integrative pediatrics," which blends traditional medicine with a holistic and nutritional approach. Oz is a highly regarded nutritional counselor and life extension specialist. I look at nutritional data in the context of the whole body and its wellness; Oz looks at wellness in the context of nutrition.

But it was our integrated approaches to medicine as a whole that attracted each of us to the other in terms of writing this book. For me, it was Oz's experience in dealing with clients who have crazy jobs and chaotic lives, who travel and who are on the move and don't necessarily have time to cook special meals for each member of the family. His practice is more about learning how nutrition can energize and recharge and revitalize health rather than prescribing checklists of what should and should not be consumed on a daily basis. For Oz, it was, as he put it, my "open-mindedness to a more holistic, complementary attitude toward health and wellness for children" that attracted him to me.

By combining our own experiences and specialized knowledge, we have created a synergistic wealth of information for parents who are desperate for answers to their children's seemingly endless medical and behavioral problems.

This book will help you understand how nutrition can dramatically, and quickly, affect a child's health—not the nutrition that's spewed out by food pyramids and calculating percentages of daily requirements, but nutrition that is based on what your body needs and how it processes various foods. This is not a diet book—it does not create rules for you to blindly follow; instead it offers new ways of thinking about food. You'll learn about the properties of food, how they work in conjunction with human biology (and how they can cause havoc in some cases). You'll discover how to make choices for your children at home, when they're at school, and when they're out with their friends at playdates and parties.

Whether you are parenting an infant, a preteen, or a child who is somewhere in between, necessity has no doubt made you become quite familiar with health issues. But it seems that as people learn more about the causes and treatments of childhood ailments, the information itself often becomes a burden. Sometimes the more parents know, the more confused they become, and with good reason. There is an astounding amount of information out there, and, unfortunately, it's often conflicting or misleading, particularly when it comes to diagnosing and treating overlapping symptoms. *The Food Cure for Kids* will help you to understand your child's immune system so that you will be better equipped to recognize and track your child's symptoms accurately and, subsequently, increase the likelihood that you will take the right steps to improve your child's health.

*The Food Cure for Kids* lets you know that it really *is* possible to take control of your child's well-being, to avoid numerous trips to the doctor's office, and to reduce those many missed days of school. The strategies in this book will help your child have more energy, more enthusiasm for daily life, fewer uncomfortable days, and fewer sleepless nights—and that's good for both of you.

*Natalie Geary, MD*

# PART I

## LAYING THE GROUNDWORK
## FOR BETTER HEALTH

# CHAPTER 1

## Is This Your Child?
## Understanding Your Constantly
## Whiny, Earache-y, Tired, Irritable,
## Stay-Home-from-School Kid

*Three-year-old Max and his mom are at the pediatrician's office—again. His nose is running like a leaky faucet. He has an ear infection for the third time this year, and it's only May. He claims that his tummy hurts, and he refused to eat any lunch, even though, as a last resort, his mom offered to take him to McDonald's. They've just come from the dermatologist's office because Max can't stop scratching the rash behind his pudgy knees. And yesterday, Max's preschool teacher told his mom that he seemed impatient and "spacey" a lot of the time.*

What is wrong with poor little Max? His mother is worried that all these maladies add up to a serious illness, while his father thinks that Max is making half of it up just to get their attention.

*Chloe is a thin, pale, four-year-old girl with wispy hair and dark circles under her eyes. Despite her low weight, her belly is slightly swollen and she sits with her mouth partially open. Her mother suspects "yet another ear infection" despite the fact that Chloe just took a course of antibiotics as recently as three weeks ago. No one in the house smokes, and their dog has been in the house since Chloe was born. As a baby she ate well, but now she is extremely picky and eats mostly pasta. She has had at least four ear infections in the past year.*

What is wrong with Chloe? Why does she always look so tired? Her mother says she barely eats but her tummy is always distended.

Do these descriptions sound familiar? Do you recognize either Max or Chloe, or maybe some combination of the two? Do you ever wonder why your little one seems to get sick so often, not with major illnesses, but with what appears to be chronic discomfort?

Perhaps your child suffers from a constant runny nose. Or a persistent cough. Maybe a skin rash that just won't go away. Or too many sleepless nights, stomachaches, or ear infections. Or worst of all, constant irritability. These common, unrelenting symptoms seem to plague our children for weeks, months, and even years at a time. Parents—who have consulted one specialist after another—are generally frustrated and the frustration is warranted; there is nothing worse than seeing your child unhealthy, uncomfortable, or simply feeling "off."

### *Is This Your Child?*

If you're not sure whether your child fits into the Max/Chloe mold, take the following quiz and answer the questions as honestly as possible.

| | Yes | No |
|---|---|---|
| 1. Does your child have "sensitive" skin, meaning his skin often gets red or blotchy? | ❑ | ❑ |
| 2. Does your child have a history of eczema (an inflammation of the skin that causes it to become red, itchy, and scaly)? | ❑ | ❑ |
| 3. Does your child ever have difficulty breathing? | ❑ | ❑ |
| 4. Does your child get frequent colds that sometimes lead to more severe symptoms? | ❑ | ❑ |
| 5. Does your child get recurrent ear infections? | ❑ | ❑ |
| 6. Does your child get recurrent sinus infections? | ❑ | ❑ |
| 7. Do your child's "seasonal allergies" seem to occur all year round? | ❑ | ❑ |

| | Yes | No |
|---|---|---|
| 8. Look at your child's eyes. Are there dark circles under her eyes, even when she has slept well? | ❏ | ❏ |
| 9. Does your child snore? | ❏ | ❏ |
| 10. Does your child normally breathe through his mouth? | ❏ | ❏ |
| 11. Is your child's stomach bloated most of the time? | ❏ | ❏ |
| 12. Does your child have foul-smelling stools (different than usual)? | ❏ | ❏ |
| 13. Does your child have difficulty concentrating or staying alert in school? | ❏ | ❏ |
| 14. Is your child a picky eater? | ❏ | ❏ |
| 15. Does your child exhibit frequent irritability that seems unprovoked? | ❏ | ❏ |

If you answered yes to eight or more of these questions, you need to keep reading this book.

It is important to consider how these different symptoms, while they may sound unconnected, are actually integrated into an overall reaction in the body. As you read the coming chapters, you will begin to realize what causes this overall reaction and how you can use simple, practical, nutritional solutions to be sure your child is on track in terms of height and weight, to help your child stay alert and focused in school, to moderate the moodiness, to reduce the number of times your child is ill, and ultimately to be sure you and your child will spend less time going to the pediatrician.

## UNDERSTANDING THE SYMPTOM COMPLEX

Have you ever found yourself on the same kind of frustrating treadmill that the parents of Max and Chloe experienced? It's not that your child is seriously ill—yet she seems to be constantly off her game. Does your child suffer from symptoms just like Max's, not to mention the coughing, the sneezing, the lack of energy, the moodiness, and the first-thing-in-the-morning-I-don't-want-to-go-to-school-today screaming fits? Perhaps you, like millions of other parents, have shuttled your child from one doctor to another and have been told to try a variety of different treatments: rounds of antibiotics for ear infections, steroid creams for eczema, breathing treatments for cough.

Those are all effective and appropriate treatments. However, when these types of noncritical illnesses and symptoms persist or recur frequently, especially when they appear as part of what is called a "symptom complex" (commonly linked symptoms that appear together), then it just might require a different approach; one that looks at and treats the whole body, not just each illness or symptom individually.

**The root cause of these disparate illnesses is more than likely nutritional imbalance.**

In fact, respiratory, skin, and gastrointestinal problems often occur together. It's time for parents and physicians alike to look at children's health from a whole new perspective and to realize that the root cause of these disparate illnesses is more than likely nutritional imbalance (for example, your child may be eating too much wheat or dairy—or both).

The illnesses and subsequent symptoms that your child is suffering from are real. Doctors are correctly diagnosing these illnesses and may be properly prescribing antibiotics or steroids to cure what's currently ailing your child. However, antibiotics and steroids will not necessarily prevent reoccurrence. This book shows you how to actually prevent these illnesses and symptoms. By making minor changes in what children eat, we can decrease their susceptibility to infection, abdominal pain, respiratory problems, lethargy, and attentional issues.

What if this symptom complex could be cured (or at least greatly reduced) by giving little Max (or Maxine) one less bowl of cereal a week, or not quite so many glasses of milk? What if there were simple nutritional changes you could make—nothing too extreme, mind you—that would recharge your child into optimum health and vitality, and would help him be much more comfortable, connected, and alert?

## INTEGRATING THE POSSIBLE AND THE PRACTICAL

This book is a guide to identifying the sources of your child's imbalances and correcting the problem with some very simple and sensible nutritional solutions. It has a unique integrative approach to health, and to helping kids stay healthy through what they eat. That's why it's set up the way it is, which may be a little different than books you're used to seeing on children's health. It's not symptom-based—the kind of book where, if your child is coughing, you look up "cough" and find suggestions for treatment. In that scenario, you wait for your child to get sick and then figure out what to do about it. In this book, you'll begin to understand how, even though the symptoms may be very different (e.g., a skin rash and a tummy ache), they're actually integrated into an overall reaction going on in the body. When you understand where this reaction originates, you can take steps before the child gets sick to prevent it from happening.

Remedies need to be both possible and practical if they're going to work. We would never recommend that you put your child on an elaborate detoxification diet, suggest that you deny him the pleasures of the real world (e.g., parties and playgrounds), or turn your home into a sterile fortress. The Cookie Monster does not have to become the Veggie Monster. It is a myth that optimum wellness requires rigidity or deprivation.

We want you to learn to look at the bigger picture, to recognize when your child is ill but also to get to know what wellness looks like—how a healthy child looks, feels, and behaves—and to watch as those problematic symptoms dissipate. The earaches will go away. Tummies won't hurt or bulge. Skin rashes will clear up. Moody little munchkins will become happy campers once more. There will be fewer and fewer trips to the pediatrician.

This book shows you that it is not only possible, but also rewarding to live in a health-conscious way without having it consume all of your time. Living in a healthy home, eating nutritiously, and raising your children in an environment beneficial to their well-being does not have to be a full-time job. It does require a working knowledge of the health factors you are dealing with, a smart analysis of the problems that exist, a little reorganization of the family's daily eating habits, a sense of perspective, and, perhaps most of all, a sense of humor.

## WHAT YOU WILL NEED TO KNOW

There are some important concepts to learn before you continue with this book. Each will be explained in more depth as the book goes on, but we're introducing them here so they will be familiar to you as you read.

**Allergy:** An allergy occurs when your immune system reacts to a foreign substance as if it was a threat to your well-being and therefore generates antibodies (infection-fighting protein molecules). An allergy is measurable via a blood test. You can't change an allergy. You may outgrow it, but at the time you are allergic, eating less of a particular food won't make you less allergic to it.

**Atopic Triad:** Atopic triad is a combination of skin, gastrointestinal, and respiratory hypersensitivities. Atopic individuals have a genetic tendency toward hypersensitive reactions to certain triggers. Triggers can be anything your body recognizes as "foreign." Triggers are different for different people; some common food triggers include nuts, shellfish, corn, wheat, and dairy. This hypersensitivity usually manifests in the form of rhinitis (a non-infectious runny nose), asthma, and/or atopic dermatitis (itchy flaking patches of sensitive skin), although how much or how little of each of these three conditions a person develops tends to vary. Studies have shown not only a significant association between these conditions but that their prevalence is increasing, particularly in children.

**Inflammatory Response:** A response of body tissues to injury or irritation, characterized by one or more of the following: pain, swelling, redness, and/or heat. This is the body's normal response to abnormal stimulation caused by disease or illness. In this book we focus on low-level chronic inflammation that occurs when the body is not in balance due to what it's being fed. It's your body's reaction to being out of balance. Most of us are somewhat inflamed almost all the time.

**Integrative Medicine:** Taking into account both Western and alternative practices, using the Eastern philosophy of looking at the whole body and wellness while still utilizing modern Western medical practices when they are indicated. It can be described as "a la carte" medicine—using whatever modality is best for a particular situation.

**Intolerance:** Intolerance is your body's inability to process the level of a particular food that you're asking your body to digest. An intolerance, or sensitivity, is not measurable, as antibodies are not produced. However, your body is not clearing the particular food out of your system very well. An intolerance is controllable, meaning if you eat less of a particular food to which you have a sensitivity, the body is better able to handle it and you will feel better.

## OUR HOPE FOR YOU

We hope after reading this book, and recognizing that the vignettes offered sound a lot like your child, you will be able to make simple yet effective modifications to your child's diet that will promote growth, alleviate the need for medicines, and encourage school performance and self-esteem. The plan here is not just to relieve symptoms, which would be nothing more than a quick fix, but instead to achieve ongoing wellness through practical changes and an openness to both Western medicine and alternative theories about medical wellness.

Our goal in writing this book was to help you identify what is ailing your child, equip you with questions to ask your doctor, and offer you solutions to try at home to restore immune balance, decrease inflammation, and improve your child's overall sense of well-being. All too often, children with intolerances and inflammation are put in "glass bubbles"—they can't eat this, they can't go there—the list of "can'ts" goes on. Our mission is to help children feel strong, safe, alert, and self-confident while still being able to participate in the real world, and to make family life easier and ease parents' worries.

Here are the main concepts that are integral to our approach:

- Children are not little adults. It's important to understand that children's nutritional needs are not just smaller versions of adults' needs. Their bodies process ingredients in different ways and cause different symptoms. For example, children's ear canals are much flatter than adults. As an adult, when you eat something that creates a lot of mucus in the body (something like dairy, which is the number one mucus-producing food), you may get a sinus infection. But you can always blow your nose. If children eat something that makes a lot of mucus, they don't always know how to blow their noses well. The mucus can pool in the flat ear canal and may not drain as well, often causing an ear infection. In addition, their immune system is more reactive so they tend to make even more mucus than adults when exposed to the same stimulants. So nutrition's impact on the interaction of anatomy, biology, and development is unique to children.

- There are many myths and misunderstandings about what children should eat. Learning about the building blocks of nutrition, including proteins, carbohydrates, and fats, as well as specific food groups such as wheat and dairy, as well as probiotics, can make a huge difference in your child's health. Part II of this book will give you all the information you need.

- It's important to understand the difference between allergies and intolerance. It's one thing if your child is allergic to peanuts, for instance, which can have dire consequences. The cause-and-effect equation is clear. It's another thing if your child has a sensitivity to wheat or dairy, which means she can tolerate the food, but not in large quantities. Your child might go to a birthday party, for instance, and have a slice of pizza and piece of birthday cake, come home and have spaghetti for dinner, wake up the next morning and have cereal for breakfast—and the next thing you know, you're back at the doctor two days later with a child who's got a respiratory infection, when what she really has is a massive wheat overload.

- For sensitivities, it's not just what a child is eating that makes the difference, but how much he is eating and in what form. Does your child have a glass of milk at every meal? We're not saying you need to cut out dairy altogether. But your child may be better off having milk in his morning cereal and then a yogurt later on in the day, or maybe his glass of milk in the evening could be half regular milk, half rice milk (a good tasting, nondairy, rice-based beverage).

- You do not have to make food look creative for children; no smiley faces with carrots or unappealing foods "disguised" to look like special treats. Is it any wonder our country is full of people with eating disorders? The whole idea is to help your kids develop a normal relationship with food.

The purpose of this book is to show you how to make doable, practical adjustments to your child's nutrition and diet. It's not necessary for a busy working mom to come home and grind her own baby food or pick vegetables from her own organic garden. Parents should be educated about what they need to pick and choose, about what's manageable and what's not manageable. You don't need to say, "My child can never have Cheetos!" You just need to know that it's like an adult drinking wine: It's perfectly okay in small doses, but you don't want to drink too much or too often. Too many parents make their kids feel like freaks by depriving them of the foods that everyone else is enjoying.

## Questions to Ask Your Child's Doctor

The best way to take advantage of your time with your child's doctor is to be as prepared as possible. Don't be shy about coming in with a list of questions; it makes it much easier on everyone if you're organized and know what information you need to discuss. Remember to limit your questions if you're there on a sick visit. Whenever possible, save the bigger questions for the well-checks because your doctor will have scheduled more time and be in a better position to really listen and talk.

Start your visit by telling the doctor, "I have a list of questions I would like to ask. When would be a good time?" That way both of you will know when to let the doctor ask you questions and when he or she will be prepared to answer yours.

Obviously the questions below and those you will find in some of the other chapters are not all relevant to every single child. Use these questions, along with the take-home points at the end of the chapters, to trigger your own questions and help you organize your thoughts before your visit.

Here are some questions you might want to ask:

- Does my child seem to have symptoms of the atopic triad?

- What are your guidelines for the use of antibiotics?

- What are your guidelines for the use of steroid creams for eczema?

- Could many of my child's ear infections, tummy aches, and mood changes be related?

- Can I talk to you about my child's diet? What changes in his diet do you think would be helpful to address his current symptoms?

- What alternatives to medicine do you believe might be helpful?

# Chapter 1 Take-Home Points

- Your child's symptoms may all be related to food intolerances and may just be an inflammatory response to whatever is triggering the reaction.

- Nutrition plays a huge role in your child's overall well-being.

- Integrative care means that we address prevention, not only disease.

- Our goals are your child's overall growth, his or her school performance and self-esteem, and keeping him or her off unnecessary medications.

It takes adults months to change their systems' balance; with children it's possible to see results within a week. Nutrition is like those levers on a stereo system that you can adjust to achieve perfect tone and pitch. What you're tinkering with are the "dials" on your child's nutritional balance, and once you find that balance, you can markedly decrease unpleasant and disparate symptoms and offer your child clarity, energy, and mood stability.

# CHAPTER 2

# An Integrative Approach: Planning for Your Child's Wellness

Why should you read this book?

Because you care about your child's health. Because you don't want your child to spend his formative years being sick and whiny and uncomfortable and unhappy and not performing to the best of his abilities. Because you don't want to spend your time and energy constantly chasing after disease; you want to stay ahead of the curve and foster wellness as much as you possibly can.

This book is based on two concepts: One is that your child is a product of the past (your past, his or her past, and the past as it applies to all human beings); in other words, we as human beings are constructed in a very particular way that makes it healthy for us to consume certain foods and unhealthy to consume others. The second concept is called integrative medicine. It is a model of healing based on wellness rather than disease, incorporating both conventional and "alternative" therapies to try to utilize the best of all practices and treatments to support each child in maintaining health and wellness in all aspects of his or her life.

By understanding this book's two main premises, you can prepare your children for a future of health, vitality, and mental clarity. We can't promise that every child will be a genius who never gets sick. But we *can* say if you follow the concepts in this book, your child will be better off. And so will you, because you will know that you have made a wise investment in your family's future.

## CONCEPT #1: WE ARE OUR PAST

If you want to peer into your child's future, you have to look to the past—the distant past, to be exact—and keep in mind that human beings are animals. In fact, we are primates. As such, we have certain fundamental requirements that must be met to ensure our survival. We must have air to breathe. We must have water to drink. And we must have food to eat.

The quality of the air we breathe and the water we drink may have declined somewhat over the thousands of years humans have existed; however, they remain substantially the same as they were 40,000 years ago. They still satisfy our genetic requirements.

The same cannot necessarily be said about food.

In fact, food has a long and extraordinary history. In order to achieve the goals of *The Food Cure for Kids,* we're going to review some of that history, because your relationship to food and its impact on your health means everything. The modern American diet has undergone a transformation of such magnitude as to constitute a new type of nourishment— if you can call it that. We'll call it *nufood.*

Our changing lifestyles and our never-ending quest for convenience have radically redefined what we eat and how we eat it. Nufood barely satisfies our genetic requirements. It does not fulfill food's primary functions of providing the mortar for building healthy bodies and brains, and the nutrients we need to live longer and to live well. It's also devoid of most of the nutritional properties that have a broad range of functions in keeping us healthy.

**Your relationship to food and its impact on your health means everything.**

We are organic bodies responsive to the natural order of the animal kingdom. As such, we must remember that *food, and specifically the nutritional value that we gain from eating it, is the central hub around which everything else (health-wise) revolves.*

### Defining "the Paleo Kid"

In defining what we call "the Paleo Kid," we begin with the premise that our bodies and minds are adapted to the world and environment of hunter/gatherers, which ended more than 10,000 years ago with the advent of agriculture. Before that time, all food was obtained by either gathering fruits, roots, tubers, nuts, seeds, herbs, and vegetables, or by hunting. And everything you could hunt was fair game for eating, every kind of animal including big and small game, fish, fowl, and eggs. Every morsel was consumed, including organs and brains. Insects and worms, good sources of protein, were also eaten. The diet was rich in what are called omega-3 essential fatty acids (see Chapter 9), which are critical to human health and terribly deficient in today's diet. The diet also provided a high volume of naturally occurring antioxidants, nutrients that protect us from many disease-causing agents.

With our modern palates and sensibilities, we're certainly not going to eat insects and worms (although kids would probably love that idea). But we do still need a rich and varied diet, high in these "native nutrients" that once allowed man to survive and thrive in a dangerous world.

Nobody expects you to feed your kids exactly and only what cavemen ate. However, were we to eat in a way closer to what our bodies adapted to through eons of evolution, we'd all be better protected from the "diseases of affluence," such as heart disease, type 2 diabetes, and many types of cancer.

Technology has provided the developed world with an unparalleled degree of comfort and convenience, taking us farther away from the foods that provide us with nutrients so essential to optimal health. We have created a consumer-oriented world of extraordinary novelty filled with nufoods that have no nutritional purpose or value. As parents, we all have the best of intentions where our kids are concerned, and we try to give them the best of everything. We would never intentionally make our kids sick. But our modern day convenience-food environment makes it so easy for us to make food choices for ourselves and our kids that may not be the healthiest options.

This is not to say that you should never allow your kids to have fast food or to have some chips now and again or to eat what's served at a birthday party. As you read the rest of this book, you'll understand how and why your children's bodies react negatively to certain foods, and what you can do—easily and practically—to mitigate these reactions.

## Small Changes Add Up to Big Results

It seems that when it comes to food, many people have difficulty changing their lifestyles and habits. That's usually because they try to make giant leaps and major shifts all at once. They cut out entire food groups. They swear off wheat altogether, or cheese, or chocolate. These tactics don't work for adults and they certainly don't work for children. What does work is making small changes every day, which will eventually add up to better health. Cut down on the number of times you serve your child bread or pasta or other wheat products in a day (see Chapter 6). Reduce, rather than eliminate, the number of dairy products in your child's diet (see Chapter 7). It's sometimes difficult to think of food in terms of anything other than what your child will actually eat. But if you really want your child to be as physically and mentally fit as possible, and to be free of the kinds of chronic complaints that turn up again and again (tummy aches, earaches, lethargy, and so on), it's important to think about what you are putting on the table as much as what your child is putting in his or her mouth. You might be surprised at what making small dietary changes can accomplish. Follow the nutritional suggestions in this book, and you will find that even as you are increasing your child's nutritional intake, you're automatically applying solutions to many of your child's health-related problems.

## CONCEPT #2: SEEING THE WHOLE CHILD

When it comes to treating children's health issues, we start from the idea of the Paleo Kid and work from there. Taking into account how the human body has evolved, we also look at what the individual child is doing right now. We use what is known as *integrative medicine* to look at the whole child.

In an ideal world, your child's mind, body, and spirit will be in balance, and any medications, treatments, or interventions will reflect the needs of the whole child. Integrative medicine literally integrates the teachings of many forms of practice, like an a la carte menu, picking and choosing the best care for each *individual* circumstance. Integrative physicians and health care practitioners like us try to avoid being too aggressive in their care, but they don't negate the need for medicine when alternatives are not appropriate. We avoid antibiotics, for example, except when they are clearly the only option. Unlike conventional Western medicine, we focus on how to strengthen and supplement the natural bodily processes to heal oneself, rather than intervening only once the patient is sick.

Children are particularly responsive to integrative care because they are fundamentally healthy and strong. Their immune systems (after six weeks of age) are generally robust, and they are forever growing and getting stronger if we feed them well, nurture them well, and protect them from toxins and stress.

### A Parent's Responsibility

Integrative care counts on parents because it is all about prevention, good nutrition, and healthy lifestyles. A child is exceptionally vulnerable to his home environment and parental practices. Parents who believe in good nutrition, healthy habits, and a healthy home give their children an express ticket to a healthier future.

Integrative doctors work with the whole person—indeed, the whole family—to look for patterns of behavior that affect health and mood, and family paradigms that work and don't work. We analyze a patient not only from the perspective of a serious illness but also from the perspective of his mood, his schedule, his family life, his school environment, and his temperament. We look at the roots of illness from all these perspectives and search for care plans that respect all the facets of each child's life. In the best of all worlds, a doctor would have ample time to spend with each and every patient and his or her entire family, and use the safest means to prevent illness, encourage wellness, and treat those diseases that could not be prevented.

### Principles of Integrative Medicine

There are several basic principles of integrative medicine, especially integrative pediatrics.

1. Prevention is better than later cure. Western medicine has always been action-oriented—focusing on reacting once a problem arises rather than educating early, watching, and waiting in an effort to lessen the likelihood that a problem will occur. Certainly there are times when intervention is lifesaving and critical, but often if the focus is on simple prevention (good nutrition, good hygiene, mental health stability), disease can be avoided.

2. Each human being is unique, and each person's response to illness and stress is therefore unique. Children are all different; even siblings respond to stressors—medical or emotional—in different ways. Illness affects each child uniquely, so the medications or treatments offered must be individualized.

3. An integrative physician or health care professional will draw from conventional and alternative therapies in order to customize the care of each patient. Relying on the wisdom of many different established practices, such as Ayurveda (an ancient Indian system of medicine that combines natural therapies with a highly individualized treatment of disease); Chinese medicine; herbal medicine; and homeopathy (a system of medicine that uses highly diluted doses from the plant, mineral, and animal kingdoms to stimulate natural defenses in the body); the integrative physician can pick and choose what will work best for the child within the context of conventional medicine.

4. The human body, especially a child's body, is inherently programmed to heal itself. Your child's immune system, unless he has an underlying disease, is innately set up to fight illness. Conventional care often disregards this, filling your child with

medications that actually suppress the body's own ability to fight disease.

5. Children are not small adults. Their bodies require thoughtful care: The challenge of pediatric medicine and integrative pediatrics is to approach and treat each child within the context of their growth and developmental stage. We must look not only at the short-term consequences of an illness and treatment plan, but also the long-term effects and the long-term goals. We must choose treatments carefully, remembering that a child is scared and suffering and vulnerable in a way that an adult is not. We want children to believe in the virtue of health maintenance.

6. Health care is a partnership between physicians and parents: As parents you must be your child's biggest advocate. This means you must speak up to your doctor—you know your child best of all, and you've spent more time with her than your doctor has in a fifteen-minute visit. Be sure to bring a list of questions to your child's doctor, and be sure that your relationship with your child's doctor is a partnership in her care, not a tutorial in parenting.

## SETTING UP YOUR CHILD'S WELLNESS PLAN

There is no doubt that what your child eats sets him up for a lifetime of health, or lack of it. Studies have shown that what children consume in the first ten years of life is more important in staving off cancer, diabetes, and other debilitating diseases than what or how they eat later in life. Healthy eating is an important part of any wellness plan for your family's future.

Now, nobody expects you to be perfect or that every meal will satisfy your child's nutritional needs. We're not trying to make you feel guilty if you and your kids go out for fast food every once in a while. We are hoping that reading this book will serve as a reminder that healthy choices can keep your kids out of the doctor's office, out of their sick beds, and back in school and at play where they should be.

> **Eat Well, Stay Well**
>
> The World Health Organization states that 65 percent of all diseases are preventable through sound nutrition.

## *What You Can Do*

As most parents eventually find out, everything works better with a plan behind it. Plans can be changed and modified as the situation requires, but starting out with a blueprint makes every task you undertake just a little easier to accomplish.

So we suggest that you make a wellness plan to ensure that your child will be as healthy as possible for as long as possible—through her formative years and on into adulthood. You want your child to thrive both physically and mentally. Although science has made many breakthrough technical advances in recent years, and for that we are very grateful, what science is now telling us is that "secrets" to good health are not very technical at all. They don't require investments of thousands of dollars or cutting-edge home gyms or exotic supplements from the mountains of the Himalayas. Science is now telling us that it is the synergy of the right foods, the right nutrients, and the right lifestyle choices that can ensure you and your children a longer, healthier, and more vital future.

> It is the synergy of the right foods, the right nutrients, and the right lifestyle choices that can ensure you and your children a longer, healthier, and more vital future.

Your wellness plan does not need to be complicated. A sample plan might include the following resolutions:

- Commit to setting a good example for your children. Where else are they going to learn what healthy eating means? There's no need to subject them to lectures on nutrition and how good spinach is for their growing bodies. Just eat some spinach yourself. Encourage them to eat it, too, and don't give up. Eventually they'll eat the spinach (or something like it) because they like to imitate what they see you do.

- Serve more fruits and veggies. Get into the habit. Let your children see that eating healthy foods isn't something we're forced to do because they're good for us; it's something we do as a matter of course. Don't make it a big deal and it won't be.

- You're the parent; they're the kids. You've got the buying power. Your children don't control what foods go in your kitchen—you do.

- Set activity examples as well as food examples. Get your kids moving and move with them. Go for age-appropriate hikes and bike rides. Or just run around the playground or backyard.

- Monitor TV, video, and computer use. Studies have shown that kids not only eat more when watching television, they eat foods that are higher in fat. You're the grown-up—let your kids know when they can watch, what they can watch, and how long they can watch it.

There are no SuperMoms or SuperDads expected here. This plan (or one you've made for yourself) works best when applied in small increments.

## Questions to Ask Your Child's Doctor

- Is my child up-to-date on all her growth and development parameters so that we can focus on wellness rather than on a particular area of concern?

- Are you, as her pediatrician, open to having discussions about a more integrative approach to my child's care? (If the answer to this is no, then you should consider how important this is to you, and whether you may want to look for a different doctor.)

- Have you ever studied integrative medicine? What is your opinion about it?

- Does my child have any underlying health concerns that would make it unsafe to alter her diet?

- Is it all right if I share with you my dietary plan for my family? Is there anything about my child that would make you concerned about my taking a stronger hand in the food my family consumes?

- Do you work with any alternative practitioners (e.g., pediatric nutritionists) who specialize in diet as a form of wellness management in children?

# Chapter 2 Take-Home Points

- This book is based on two concepts: One is that we as human beings are constructed in a very particular way that makes it healthy for us to consume certain foods and unhealthy to consume others. The second concept is called integrative medicine, a model of healing that is based on wellness rather than disease and incorporates both conventional and "alternative" therapies to try to utilize the best of all practices and treatments to support each child in maintaining health and wellness in all aspects of his or her life.

- Your relationship to food and its impact on your health means everything.

- We must always remember our roots: We are organic bodies responsive to the natural order of the animal kingdom. As such, we must also remember that *food, and the nutritional value we get from it, is the central hub around which everything else (health-wise) revolves.*

- We have created a consumer-oriented world filled with nufoods that have no nutritional purpose or value. The modern day convenience-food environment makes it so easy for us to make nutritional choices for ourselves and our kids that may not be the healthiest choices we can make.

- What works best is making small changes every day rather than trying to enact drastic change all at once.

- Integrative pediatrics looks at the whole child and combines the teachings of many different practices to create the best care plan for each *individual* circumstance and child.

- Integrative care's focus on prevention relies on parents to help set a strong foundation of good nutrition and healthy habits to ensure a healthier future for their children.

- Make a wellness plan to ensure that your children will be as healthy as possible for as long as possible There are several simple steps you can follow:

  - Commit to setting a good example for your children.

  - Serve more fruits and veggies.

  - You're the parent; they're the kids. Your children don't control what foods go in your cupboards—you do.

  - Set activity examples as well as food examples. Get your kids moving and move with them.

  - Monitor TV, video, and computer use. Let your kids know when they can watch, what they can watch, and how long they can watch it.

In the next chapter, you will see just how much the food we eat affects every system in our body, from our hormones to our metabolism to our ability to think and focus. It especially affects how we defend ourselves against all those nasty germs and toxins with the help of our remarkable immune system.

# CHAPTER 3

# Immune System 101:
# The Body's (Sometimes Overly Sensitive) Defense System

In an exhibition called "Bodies," which has traveled the world since 2005, you can view actual human specimens that have been preserved—some full bodies, some sets of bones, muscles, and organs—all of which are fascinating and beautiful. Unless you're a medical professional, it's not often that you get the chance to get a close-up look into the human body's complex inner workings. Not only is the exhibit educational, it also makes you stop and think about just how fragile and vulnerable a life force we are, and how amazing it is that we manage to survive at all.

One of the reasons we do survive, often against great odds, is the body's incredible built-in defense mechanism known as the immune system. The immune system is where we house our army of cellular warriors that do their best to keep foreign invaders away from our vital organs and to kill those invaders that do get past their best defenses. Those invaders may come from surfaces we touch, from the air we breathe, and/or from the food we eat. For the purposes of this book, we're mostly concerned with how the immune system interacts with the food we eat and drink.

The kinds of food we eat have a direct, chemical-based effect on us from the first bite we take in the morning to the last snack before bedtime. Food modifies our hormones. It can improve or impair our metabolism. It can increase or decrease our energy levels. It can strengthen or weaken our concentration and brain performance. For instance, yogurt contains probiotics, friendly bacteria that live in our "gut" and not only help with our digestion, but also help keep our immune systems functioning properly as well. And scientists now know that there is a direct connection between food—specifically the nutrients derived from food—and a healthy or compromised immune system. In order to appreciate that relationship, it's important to first understand the immune system and how it works.

### FOREIGN BODIES AND ANTIBODIES

The immune system is the body's defense against infectious organisms and other invaders. If everything is going well, you never notice your immune system at work. It does its job quietly and efficiently, and you feel fit and healthy. You only notice the immune system (even though you may not consciously know that's what it is) when something has gone wrong—when, for instance, a cut gets infected, glands get swollen, or your throat becomes painfully raw and scratchy. That happens because we are bombarded every day by millions of bacteria, viruses, microbes (tiny living organisms), toxins, and parasites—better known in lay terms as "germs"—that have evolved to survive and reproduce within our bodies. The whole immune system is evolutionary, meaning that germs are getting better and better at fighting us, and we (in theory) are getting better at fighting them. The bacteria that have evolved the most are the ones that have survived to better invade our immune systems.

**We are bombarded every day by millions of bacteria, viruses, microbes (tiny living organisms), toxins, and parasites—better known in lay terms as "germs"—that have evolved to survive and reproduce within our bodies.**

Germs come in through cuts in the skin, via insect bites, through the air we breathe, and in and on the food we eat. If you get sick, these organisms are winning the war. If you don't fall ill, the immune system is prevailing.

The immune system protects you in three basic ways:

1.  It creates a barrier that prevents germs from entering your body.

2.  If germs do enter your body, it goes after them before they can reproduce.

3.  If they do reproduce, the immune system fights to get rid of them.

If a foreign substance (known as an *antigen*) invades your body, it triggers a series of steps known as the immune response, which involves a network of cells, tissues, and organs that work together to protect the body.

Some of the most important warriors of your immune system army are your white blood cells, which start off in bone marrow as stem cells (generic cells that can form into many different types of cells). There are many different types of white blood cells in your body, but they all have the same mission: to move around the body and destroy, immobilize, or neutralize disease-causing enemy invaders. One of the most effective weapons they use to capture these cells is called an *antibody*. These are Y-shaped proteins that respond to specific antigens. In simple terms, the antibody binds to a virus or a bacterium and stops it from moving through healthy cell walls.

### Immunity Times Three

Humans have three types of immunity:

**Innate Immunity:** This is immunity that "comes with the package"—we're born with it. It includes the natural barriers we have to protect ourselves, like the skin and the mucous membranes that line the nose, throat, and gastrointestinal tract, which are our first line of defense against invaders.

**Adaptive Immunity:** This type of immunity involves lymphocytes, white blood cells that allow the body to recognize previous invaders and help destroy them. That's why once you get chickenpox, you don't get it again. It's also how vaccination works. Particular antigens are introduced to the body in small amounts. This signals the body to make antibodies that are designed specifically to fight any future invasions of that particular antigen.

**Passive Immunity:** Passive immunity is temporary immunity that comes from an outside source and lasts a short time. For example, all babies have antibodies from their mothers, which give them short-term protection from diseases to which their mothers have been exposed.

## THE BIG CONFUSION: BACTERIA OR VIRUS?

Although the immune system is amazingly efficient, it isn't perfect. If it was, no one would ever get sick. In many cases, even though the immune system can't prevent you from developing an illness, it can help you recover in a timely manner. You may not be able to ward off the common cold, but a healthy immune system can shorten its lifespan and severity. You can help your child's immune system stay strong and fight illness by educating yourself about certain terms and conditions. One of the most important things to know is the difference between bacterial and viral infections.

- **Bacterial infections** are caused by bacteria, microscopic single-celled living organisms that reproduce by dividing. They can reproduce quickly, and may be capable of causing disease. They can be found on both living and nonliving substances; they can, for instance, grow on doorknobs and countertops as well as on the food you eat. Bacteria are the most abundant of all organisms. There are approximately ten times more bacterial cells than any other kind of cells in the entire body, with large numbers of bacteria on the skin and in the gut. The vast majority of bacteria in the body are rendered harmless by the protective effects of the immune system. Some bacteria are beneficial, as you will learn in Chapter 10 on probiotics.

- **Viral infections** are caused by viruses, capsules of genetic material that can reproduce only inside a living host, such as a person, a plant, or an animal. The DNA in the virus allows it to make copies of itself only when inside the host. A virus is so small (much smaller than a bacterium) that it can't carry all the DNA it needs to replicate itself, so it takes over some of the host's cell machinery to generate new virus parts. Eventually, the host cell dies and bursts, freeing the new virus particles to infect other cells.

Why is it important to know the difference? Because these two types of infection cannot be treated in the same way, nor do they respond to the same medications. In America, most people seem to feel that if a person gets sick, a pill will take care of the problem. This assumption is especially true when that person is your child. That's probably because none of us wants to see our kids suffer, so we want the quickest possible remedy. Unfortunately, we can't always get what we want.

Bacterial infections are treated with antibiotics, chemicals that kill the bacteria cells but do not affect the cells that make up your body. They are usually effective at clearing up bacterial infections. However, they lose effectiveness over time. Bacteria can mutate, and then the specific antibiotic designed to fight it no longer works. Taking antibiotics when you don't need to can lead to antibiotic-resistant germs; this is one reason you don't want to use antibiotics too often. If you don't take antibiotics when they are needed, the infection may clear up by itself. On the other hand, it may continue to get worse and could lead to serious consequences such as permanently damaged tissue, severe illness, and in extreme cases, death.

**Taking antibiotics when you don't need to can lead to antibiotic-resistant germs.**

In the case of viral infections, there are a few antiviral medications for certain types of viral infections, but for the most part, you simply have to wait out a virus.

### MOMMY, WHAT'S MAKING MY EAR ACHE?

A vast amount of confusion exists when it comes to earaches. That's because they can be caused by both bacteria and viruses. A doctor can't tell if it's a bacterial or viral infection just by looking into your child's ear. The doctor should be asking you questions in order to make a diagnosis. First, she might ask if your child has been vaccinated, and if so, which vaccinations he or she has had (it's important to keep this information handy, especially if you're taking your child to a doctor she hasn't seen before). If so, that means your child has been vaccinated against the bacteria that cause earaches. The doctor should also ask how long your child has had the earache. Bacterial infections usually last longer than viral infections. If your kid has had an earache for more than three days, it's probably bacterial. In that case, your child should be put on antibiotics. However, in an otherwise healthy child who has been vaccinated, 85 percent of ear infections are viral—meaning he or she does not need antibiotics and should be feeling better within three or four days.

---

### Does My Child Really Need an Antibiotic?

Most earaches do not require antibiotics, but sometimes doctors prescribe them anyway just to be "on the safe side." That's not always the best thing for your child. You should ask your doctor several questions to help determine the best course of action:

- What is the likelihood, given that my child has been immunized, that it is a bacterial infection?

- When was the last time you gave him antibiotics?

- What would be the harm in waiting for forty-eight hours before starting my child on an antibiotic, giving her Tylenol for pain, lots of fluids, and rest in the meantime? If my child is getting worse, I will call you before then.

---

## THE MUCUS-FOOD-IMMUNE CONNECTION

Gross as it may be to some of us, we can't have a discussion of kids and the immune system without talking about mucus. If you're a parent, you're probably quite familiar with mucus—or what you think mucus is. Most parents think it's what stuffs up a child's nose. And it is—but it's so much more as well. Mucus is actually found throughout the body. It's a thick, lubricating fluid produced by the mucous membranes that line the respiratory, digestive, urinary, and reproductive tracts. It serves as a barrier against infection and, in the digestive tract, moistens food, making it easier to swallow.

Mucous membranes line body cavities such as the mouth and stomach. These structures secrete saliva and hydrochloric acid, chemicals that destroy bacteria. If antigens pass through these defenses, a variety of white blood cells tries to destroy them. Mucus is especially important for children, because it supports their growth process. Just like plants need moisture to grow, so do young bodies, and much of that moisture comes from mucus. That's why mucus production is heaviest during the first twelve years of a child's life. It begins to slow down during the teen years, usually stabilizes during adult years, and sometimes begins to dry out as we get into seniorhood.

**An overproduction of mucus can actually be triggered by a nutritional imbalance.**

If your child is constantly getting colds or the flu, or has asthma or other respiratory conditions, it may be because his or her mucus factory is working overtime and there is a surplus being produced. That's not a good thing, and here's why: If your body is generating too much mucus, it's like having a stagnant pond in your backyard. Stagnant water allows bacteria to thrive. If you have excess mucus sitting in your upper respiratory space—your nose, your sinuses, your ears—it's like a feeding ground for bacteria. You're creating your own inner petri dish in which bacteria will grow and reproduce. What many parents don't know is that an overproduction of mucus can actually be triggered by a nutritional imbalance.

Too much mucus is an open invitation to infection. Not only that, kids who consistently have a head full of mucus often feel lethargic and groggy, as if their head is in a vise. They walk around with their mouths open all the time, spaced out and glassy-eyed. They're exhausted because their immune system is totally out of whack. Less mucus means more energy, clearer thinking, and improved appetite.

## Why Are Ear Infections So Common?

Does your child seem to get an ear infection every time he or she gets a cold? When another child in day care or school has an ear infection, does your youngster get one, too? This fairly common occurrence is largely due to anatomy. As we learned in Chapter 1, a child's ear canal (also known as the eustachian tube), a passageway that sits in the back of the throat and leads to the middle ear cavity, is much narrower and flatter than an adult's. This tube helps drain extra fluid from the middle ear. When a child has a cold, swelling in the nose may impede drainage. Germs (either viruses or bacteria) can enter the middle ear and cause an infection. The infection results in increased fluid in the ear and can cause pain, fever, and irritability. As you age, that canal gets wider and steeper. That's why as a small child you are more prone to ear infections, and as you get older and your sinuses develop, you are more prone to sinus infections. When the tube is still narrow and flat, fluid (mucus) just sits there and becomes a good medium for bacterial growth or viral infection. Some middle school–age children whose tubes have not yet gotten steep enough still get ear infections. But for the most part, by the time a child is twelve to fourteen years old, ear infections will have become a thing of the past.

### Mucus-Producing Foods

Certain foods tend to trigger the body into producing more mucus than other foods. Dairy foods, especially milk, cheese, cream, and butter, produce the most mucus. That means that foods made with these items—such as pizza, ice cream, grilled cheese sandwiches, cereal with milk, and so on—may result in respiratory problems for your child. Bread, which is made with wheat, can also cause an increase in mucus production. Both milk and bread have large protein molecules (casein in milk, gluten in wheat), glue-like substances that bind their molecules together, which make them difficult to digest and can cause irritation in the body.

Here are some examples of foods that produce mucus and foods that don't:

| Mucus-Forming Foods | Non-Mucus-Forming Foods | |
|---|---|---|
| All dairy products | Asparagus | Broccoli |
| Bananas | Cantaloupe | Apples |
| Meat | Endive | Cucumbers |
| Processed foods | Fruit Juices | Onions |
| Saturated fats | Grapes | Lettuce |
| Sugar | Lemons | Pears |
| Wheat | Limes | Avocado |
| Potatoes | Olive Oil | Quinoa |
| | Papaya | Carrots |
| | Tomatoes | Mushrooms |
| | Watercress | Oranges |
| | Watermelons | Pineapple |
| | Chamomile Tea | |

Does that mean you need to cut out mucus-forming foods altogether? No, of course not. But you might want to cut down on the amount of these types of foods you feed your child on any given day. You might not want to feed your child a breakfast of milk and cereal, followed by a lunch of macaroni and cheese, and then pizza for dinner with ice cream for dessert. (Check out Chapter 7, "Let's Get Specific: Dairy," to find alternative products for lessening a dairy overload.) How much is too much? There's no cookie-cutter answer to that. If your child is prone to colds, flu, asthma, or earaches, cut back on these foods and see what happens. It may be that one less serving a day will do the trick. If your child is more sensitive, one serving a week may be all he or she can tolerate.

---

### A Spoonful of Sugar

Sugar may be making your child overweight—but it may also be making her sick. Studies have shown that eating or drinking 100 grams (8 tablespoons) of sugar can reduce white blood cells' ability to kill germs by 40 percent. Eight tablespoons may sound like a lot, but it's the equivalent of two and a half 12-ounce cans of soda, not an outrageous amount for a child to consume in a day. The immune-suppressing effect of sugar starts less than thirty minutes after ingestion and can last as long as five hours.

---

## IT'S ALL ABOUT REACTIVITY AND BALANCE

The immune system is, by nature, reactive—more defensive than offensive. In other words, it is in a constant state of readiness but doesn't take action until it senses some kind of disturbance.

In some people, the immune system doesn't work as it should. In people who have AIDS, for instance, the immune system loses most of its ability to react, and it no longer produces the fighter cells needed to keep the body healthy and infection-free. On the other hand, some people's immune systems are so hyperactive that they perceive the body's own tissues as foreign and attack them. These people can develop auto-immune diseases like rheumatoid arthritis and lupus.

The immune system of a child is virginal in that it has not yet been introduced to the many different germs and toxins adults process easily every day. Children's glands, lymph nodes (small bean-shaped tissue masses that act as filters of impurities in the body), tonsils, adenoids, and turbinates (nasal passages) are easily hypertrophied, which means they get really large in response to foreign invaders. As we get older, our immune systems are not as reactive.

We don't want the immune system to be overreactive, nor do we want it to be underreactive. We want it to be just right. We want a stable response, meaning that it's being stimulated in response to appropriate stimuli like bacteria or viruses. It's not making too much mucus; it's not making too many antibodies or no antibodies at all. The point is to get the body into balance and keep it there so that the immune system can save its energy to fight real infection.

**We don't want the immune system to be overreactive, nor do we want it to be underreactive.**

One of the things that can be most confusing about an imbalance in the immune system is that it causes seemingly unrelated symptoms. It creates the earache/tummy ache/fatigue/irritability/I-don't-want-to-go-to-school syndrome so prevalent in children these days. That is because there are mutually intersecting systems within the body that seem to be distinct, yet they profoundly influence one another in ways that either maintain or disrupt the balance. This concept of balance and interaction, once appreciated, enables you to correct and adjust your child's health in subtle and meaningful ways.

## IMMUNITY BOOSTERS

If you want to keep your kids' immune system in tip-top shape, there is nothing better than a balanced diet. However, there are certain foods you can serve that are particularly good for improving immune system function:

- Whole grains, such as brown rice, quinoa, oats, and barley

- Green leafy vegetables, such as spinach, kale, and collard greens

- Orange vegetables, such as carrots, sweet potatoes, squash, and pumpkin

- Proteins, such as salmon, trout, tuna, and red meat

- Yogurt that contains probiotics

- Green tea

### Had Some Quinoa Lately?

Quinoa (*kee-nwa*) is one of the tastiest, healthiest foods you've probably never heard of. It is an amino acid–rich seed that has a fluffy, creamy, slightly crunchy texture and a somewhat nutty flavor when cooked. Even though it's usually included in the category of whole grains, it is really a relative of leafy green vegetables like spinach and Swiss chard. Quinoa is high in fiber and is a complete protein, meaning it has all nine amino acids (see Chapter 8), and is an excellent source of minerals including magnesium, copper, and iron. It's been around for many hundreds of years and was once considered "the gold of the Incas." It's easy to prepare and can be found in many supermarkets and in virtually every health food store in the country.

### *Exercise and the Immune System*

Another great way to boost your kids' immune systems is to get them moving. More and more, research is finding a link between moderate, regular exercise and a strong immune system. Studies have shown that exercise has been linked to a positive immune system response and a temporary boost in the production of macrophages, the cells that attack bacteria. It is believed that regular, consistent exercise can lead to substantial benefits in immune system health over the long-term. During moderate exercise immune cells circulate through the body more quickly and are better able to kill bacteria and viruses (too much intense exercise can have the opposite effect). After exercise ends, the immune system generally returns to normal within a few hours, but consistent, regular exercise seems to make these changes last longer.

### *Sleep and the Immune System*

What happens when you and your family go on vacation and your kids run around like crazy, go to sleep later, and get up earlier than they usually do? More than likely, they get sick as soon as you get home (if not sooner). Or what happens when your child stays up into the wee hours to study for an important, stress-producing exam? You can bet he'll be home from school the day after the test with a cold or the flu.

**Sleep promotes the immune system and the immune system promotes sleep.**

When you sleep, your body creates cytokines, small proteins released by cells that, among other things, help fight off infections. When you don't get enough sleep, fewer of these cytokines are produced, and your chances of getting sick increase. Then an interesting phenomenon occurs: When you do get sick, the body produces more cytokines, which act like sedatives to help you get the sleep you need (which is why you get so tired when you're not feeling well). So sleep promotes the immune system and the immune system promotes sleep.

# Questions to Ask Your Child's Doctor

- Is my child getting more than the usual number of childhood infections? If so, what suggestions do you have for preventing further infections?

- If my child has an infection, what should I look for before starting antibiotics? How long is it safe to observe before I bring her in or call you for an appointment?

- Would you recommend (or object to) trying any alternatives to antibiotics first (e.g., garlic oil for ears, chamomile tea for respiratory mucus, zinc for sore throats)?

# Chapter 3 Take-Home Points

- The immune system is the body's defense mechanism, protecting us against germs that come from surfaces we touch, air we breathe, and food we eat and drink.

- If a foreign substance (known as an antigen) invades your body, it triggers the immune response, which involves a network of cells, tissues, and organs that work together to protect the body.

- It is important to know the difference between bacterial and viral infections. Bacteria are microscopic single-celled living organisms that reproduce by dividing. They can reproduce quickly, and may be capable of causing disease. Viruses are capsules of genetic material that can reproduce only inside a living host, such as a person, a plant, or an animal.

- Bacterial infections can be treated with antibiotics; viral infections cannot.

- If your child is constantly getting colds or the flu, or has asthma or other respiratory conditions, it may be because his or her mucus factory is working overtime and there is a surplus being produced. Too much mucus is a breeding ground for bacteria.

- Dairy and wheat products are the biggest mucus-producing foods. Too many servings of foods like pizza, ice cream, cheese, and milk may cause overproduction of mucus, which young bodies cannot eliminate, thereby creating bacterial breeding grounds.

- It's all about balance. You don't want your child's immune system to be overreactive, yet you don't want it to be underreactive either. Maintaining your child's healthy immune system balance will help reduce instances of colds and flu, improve school performance and concentration, and keep her out of the doctor's office.

One of the most obvious signs of an out-of-balance immune system is a food allergy or intolerance. This can happen when the system over-reacts to particular antigens that for most people cause no reaction at all. The next chapter will fill you in on the differences between allergies and intolerances, how they affect your children, and what you can do about them.

CHAPTER 4

# It's Probably Not Allergies:
# Allergy vs. Intolerance

*When Lydia brought three-year-old Rowan in to see me, she also brought in a large handful of tissues, which she used to wipe Rowan's constantly running nose. She told me that Rowan had not been sleeping well for weeks, and that for the past three days he'd been complaining about tummy aches. Worst of all, as his mother put it, "My precious good-natured baby has turned into a cranky, moody sulker."*

*In my pediatric practice, I am regularly asked to see children with low-grade but unrelenting symptoms. Their parents are either embarrassed to bring their child in because there's nothing terribly wrong, or they've already been to see several specialists who can find no cause for their child's discomfort and seem to dismiss it out of hand. Parents are understandably frustrated. As a parent myself, I know there are few things worse than seeing your child uncomfortable for no apparent reason.*

*—From Dr. Geary's files*

Given the recent proliferation of news articles, TV coverage, and parent newsletters about childhood allergies, many parents may assume that chronic discomfort means that their child has developed allergies. However, that assumption is often misguided. In fact, most children who have persistent runny noses, rashes, gastrointestinal illnesses, and other chronic conditions do not have true allergies at all. They may have what is known as a *sensitivity*, or a food intolerance.

This is the crux of this book. Most kids do not have allergies. And if they do, they have to avoid that food at all costs (no peanuts, ever!). If they have an intolerance, they can eat nuts (or whatever food is causing the problem) once in a while, maybe even more often than that, but not all in one day. It's about the quantity and frequency of exposure. It doesn't mean you have to eliminate any food from your child's diet; it means that you (or the child, depending on his or her age) have to keep track of how often your child is con- **Most kids** suming the food and how much of it she is consuming. If **do not have** your child is eating Honey Nut Cheerios for breakfast, a **allergies.** Snickers candy bar for a snack, a peanut butter and jelly sandwich for lunch, and pecan-crusted fried chicken for dinner, she may not break out in hives or have difficulty breathing. But the next day, she just might have a crampy stomachache or be inexplicably irritable, both probably due to the fact that she went over her sensitivity limit by eating all those nut-based foods in one day.

So you can see why food-related allergies and intolerances require different nutritional approaches. The rest of this chapter will explain the difference between the two, and what to do if you suspect your child has either.

### WHAT IS AN ALLERGY?

True allergic reactions cause the body's immune system to develop antibodies against what it perceives to be a foreign invader. This "invader" is usually a protein. The first time you ingest this protein, the immune system responds by creating specific antibodies called immunoglobulin E, or IgE. Every time you eat this food again, the body sends out IgE antibodies and other chemicals, including histamine (which is why some allergy medications are called antihistamines). And although antibodies are usually protective, IgE antibodies can cause a broad variety of inflammatory reactions. These reactions can range anywhere from mild to extreme; in the worst cases, allergies can be deadly. Symptoms of a food allergy may include:

- Anaphylaxis (a sudden, severe, potentially life-threatening allergic reaction)

- Chest pain

- Diarrhea

- Hives

- Itchy skin

- Nausea

- Rash

- Shortness of breath

- Stomach pains

- Swelling of the airways to the lungs

- Watery eyes

Allergies are measurable in the blood, and there is a whole subset of people who are truly allergic. Reactions can be triggered by even a very small amount of the food; people who are allergic to a particular food are advised to avoid that food completely.

Allergic disorders include:

- **Allergies:** You can be allergic to almost anything in the environment, such as pollen or dust mites; you can have seasonal allergies like hay fever; you may react negatively to specific medications or drugs; toxins that come from insect bites and bee stings can bring on reactions; and finally, foods can cause the body to produce the IgE antibodies that signal allergy.

- **Asthma:** Asthma is a breathing disorder that involves an allergic reaction in the lungs. Certain allergens (such as pollen, mold, animal dander, and so on) can trigger breathing tubes in the lungs to become narrowed, making it more difficult for a person to breathe. Asthma can be mild, requiring an at-home inhaler, or it can be so severe as to be life-threatening.

- **Eczema:** This is an itchy skin rash also known as atopic dermatitis. It is not necessarily caused by an allergic reaction, but often occurs in young children and adolescents who have allergies, hay fever, or asthma.

### *The Usual Suspects*

No one knows exactly why some people are allergic to certain foods. Heredity does play a factor, although it is not the whole story. Some experts believe that babies who are bottle-fed are more likely to develop certain allergies. Another theory says that introducing foods such as citrus fruits, cow's milk, and wheat too soon into an infant's diet may cause allergies to these substances.

It is possible to be allergic to any food. However, there are eight foods that account for 90 percent of all allergic reactions:

- Milk

- Eggs

- Peanuts

- Fish

- Shellfish

- Soy

- Wheat

- Tree nuts (like cashews, walnuts, pecans, and almonds)

Milk and egg allergies are more common in very young children and are often outgrown as they get older. Peanut, fish, and shellfish allergies are more common in older children and adults and tend to last for many years or for life.

As of January 2006, all food products must clearly say on the package if they contain any of the foods that are responsible for most allergies. If you have a child with true allergies, get used to reading *all* food labels, as allergens can turn up in unlikely places. Candy bars, for instance, may contain corn, wheat, soy, or eggs . . . and the ingredient may not always be spelled out clearly. The product may list gluten as an ingredient, for example, which comes from wheat, or casein, which is a milk protein. It pays to be educated where allergies are concerned.

## Avoiding Allergic Reactions—One Food at a Time

A 2008 study in the journal *Pediatrics* reported that about 6 percent of babies have food allergies by the end of their first year. In order to detect possible food allergies in your infant, it's best to introduce him to one food at a time. Here are some simple tips for introducing new foods to your baby:

- Start with a single-ingredient food such as a single-grain infant cereal or pureed meats.

- Although many experts say you should stay with this food for two to four days before introducing a new food, we believe you should wait five to seven days. If there is no reaction, like a rash or upset stomach, your child is probably not allergic. A reaction can actually manifest up to seven days after ingesting the food; if you introduce a second food within that week and the child reacts, you won't know which food caused the reaction. This is especially true for children who have a family history of allergies or food issues. Our philosophy is: Children have a lifetime to try new foods. What's the rush?

- If your baby does react, discontinue that food and contact your pediatrician.

- Every week, introduce a single-ingredient fruit or vegetable and watch for reactions.

- Once your baby has adapted to a variety of single-ingredient foods, it is okay to combine them. It's not okay to introduce a mixed variety of things he's never had before. Once you know that he's tolerated bananas and pears, for instance, you can then give him bananas and pears mixed together. You shouldn't feed him bananas and strawberries until he's been introduced to each separately.

### *Allergies Are on the Rise*

In 2007, the National Center for Health Statistics (part of the Centers for Disease Control and Prevention) reported that about 4 percent of children under the age of eighteen in the United States—about three million children—had food allergies, an 18 percent increase since 1997.

No one knows exactly why this is happening, although there are several theories. One is called the "hygiene hypothesis," which says that people in industrialized countries are living in increasingly sterilized environments; as a result their immune systems don't have to fight as many infections and thus don't develop as many antibodies to fend off diseases and allergies. Other theories mention eating more processed foods with ingredients the body doesn't necessarily recognize, as well as the increase in eating out, where you don't have total control over what you're eating.

If you think your child is allergic to a specific food, you should visit your pediatrician. The doctor will want to know exactly what precipitated the reaction, and he or she will probably ask you a series of questions regarding the child's food history. Be prepared for this visit by answering the questions below before you get to the doctor's office:

How old is your child? _____

What food caused the reaction? _____

How much of the food did the child eat? _____

Has the child eaten this food before? _____

What was the reaction (nausea, vomiting, rash, etc.)? _____
_____

Describe the reaction as specifically as possible: If it was a rash, was it a rash on the trunk or a rash on the face? Was it hives? Was it little red dots? If possible, take a picture. The symptom may be gone by the time you get to the doctor. _____
_____
_____

How soon after eating did the reaction occur? _____

Was the child eating any other foods at the time? _____

What else was going on at the time? (Was the child ill? Was she running around or exercising vigorously? Was he on any medication?)

_____

_____

### Testing for Allergies

There are a number of different ways to test for food allergies, but there are two that are most common:

- **Skin test.** In this test, a drop of the allergen in question is placed on the skin and the skin is then scratched or pricked with a needle. The testing is not painful, and generally there is no bleeding involved since the needle only scratches the surface of the skin. Results will show on the skin in a matter of minutes. A skin test is helpful in uncovering hidden food allergies, but it has a high incidence of false positives, meaning the skin test is likely to show that your child is allergic to a food when he really is not.

- **Blood test.** Radioallergosorbent testing (RAST) involves measuring specific allergic antibodies in a person's blood. While skin testing can give a sense, based on the size of the reaction, of whether a person is truly allergic to the food, RAST actually measures the amount of allergic antibody to the food. RAST is more expensive than skin testing, and it takes several days to get results.

Neither one of these tests is totally reliable. That is, a test may indicate that you are allergic to a food that further tests may show you are not allergic to (false positive results). And you might get a false negative result (meaning the test shows you not to be allergic when you really are) if you are on an antihistamine such as Claritin or Zyrtec or have recently had a viral infection that suppresses the immune system.

The best method of detection is for you to be as observant as possible, to record any reactions your child has to particular foods, and then to discuss these with your pediatrician. It's important to note that many children with food allergies become tolerant to those foods over time. This is most likely to happen with allergies to cow's milk, eggs, wheat, and soybeans. It's least likely to happen with peanut, tree-nut, and seafood allergies.

## WHAT IS A FOOD INTOLERANCE?

There are many people who are not allergic but who do have problems with certain foods. If you or your child is in that category, it might be because of a food intolerance. A food intolerance is not the same as a food allergy. An intolerance is not immune mediated—in other words, it does not cause your body to generate antibodies against a food. It is caused by a problem in the way the body processes a particular food or food additive. For example, people with lactose intolerance often have stomach pains or diarrhea after consuming milk products, but this is caused by a lack of lactose enzymes or metabolites, rather than an immune response (for more information on lactose intolerance, see Chapter 7). And, importantly, food intolerance does not lead to anaphylaxis (allergic shock reaction) or require that you completely avoid the particular food. An intolerance means that you will feel better if you avoid the food—your belly will be less bloated, your stool less erratic, you energy level better—but you are not going to end up in the emergency room if you eat the food by accident.

> An intolerance means that you will feel better if you avoid the food—your belly will be less bloated, your stool less erratic, you energy level better—but you are not going to end up in the emergency room if you eat the food by accident.

According to the Food Allergy and Anaphylaxis Network, a non-profit information and advocacy group, approximately twelve million Americans (one in twenty-five) suffer from food allergies. One in seventeen children age three and under has a food allergy. Food intolerances are much more common. Along with allergies, reported cases of gluten (wheat) and lactose (milk) intolerance have increased over the past decade, perhaps as each condition has garnered more attention and awareness. In addition, the amount of chemicals and other irritants that can be found in foods today simply didn't exist in the past, and our developing immune systems may be flooded and overwhelmed, hyperstimulated, and looking for relief. Just like a newborn that gets hiccups from overstimulation of the nervous system, a growing child's immune system can get over-triggered by early or overwhelming exposures to unfamiliar foods and additives and become hypersensitive.

Most children do not have hard-core allergies—what they have is the hypersensitivity described above. This means the body does not recognize these substances as foreign, so it doesn't produce antibodies. But it's like having mud in the pipes: It doesn't cause a complete halt, but it clogs the system.

Intolerances are different than allergies in many other ways as well. First, they are more variable than allergies. Food allergies can be triggered by even a tiny amount of the food, and the same or similar symptoms occur each time the food is ingested. True allergies are predictable and generate stereotypic immune responses such as hives, wheezing, and more severe reactions that may require emergency room visits. Intolerances are more fluid and changeable. There are no skin or blood tests for food intolerances. Symptoms don't usually show up unless you eat a large portion of the problem food or eat it frequently. Intolerances usually produce less dramatic problems than allergies, such as:

- Bloating

- Cramps

- Diarrhea

- Excess mucus production

- Fatigue

- Gas

- Headaches

- Heartburn

- Irritability or nervousness

- Nausea

- Stomach pain

- Vomiting

### *Keeping a Food Diary*

If your child suffers from one or more of the food intolerance symptoms, it's a good idea to look into what might be causing or exacerbating these symptoms. You probably already have some sense of your child's daily eating habits, but the questionnaire provided below will help you take an organized inventory. This inventory is comprised of a food diary and a sleep diary, which provide a written record of your child's sleep habits, including naps, and everything your child eats—all foods, beverages, condiments, snacks, and candies. Using these tools you (and your pediatrician) will be able to analyze the data to determine what kind of reactions your child has, what system of the body it refers to, and what the information you've gathered says about potential triggers.

Food Diary Week of _____

| Day: | Food | Reaction Time | Description of Reaction |
|---|---|---|---|
| Breakfast<br>Time: | | | |
| Snack<br>Time: | | | |
| Lunch<br>Time: | | | |
| Snack<br>Time: | | | |
| Dinner<br>Time: | | | |
| Snack<br>Time: | | | |

Example

| Day:<br>SUNDAY | Food | Reaction Time | Reaction Description |
|---|---|---|---|
| **Breakfast**<br>Time: 7:00 a.m. | 2 eggs, bacon,<br>toast w/butter,<br>glass of milk | 8:00 a.m. | Mild stomachache |
| **Snack**<br>Time: 10:45 a.m. | 6 oz. container<br>blueberry yogurt | | None |
| **Lunch**<br>Time: 12:30 p.m. | 2 frozen waffles<br>w/maple syrup<br>& butter, glass<br>of milk, 2 Oreo<br>cookies | 2:30 p.m. | Mild stomachache,<br>bloating, gas |
| **Snack**<br>Time: 3:30 p.m. | 1 6.75 oz. box<br>cherry Juicy Juice | | None |

| Day: SUNDAY | Food | Reaction Time | Reaction Description |
|---|---|---|---|
| **Dinner**<br>Time: 6:00 p.m. | Chicken fingers, corn w/butter, broccoli florets, 1 biscuit w/butter, 1 container Juicy Juice | | None |
| **Snack**<br>Time: 8:15 p.m. | 3 Oreo cookies, 1 glass chocolate milk | 9:15 p.m. | Stomach cramps, diarrhea |

The sample diary above indicates that the child in question may be suffering from an intolerance to either wheat or dairy (or possibly both). With this information, your next step might be to cut down on milk consumption for the next two weeks and see if that makes any difference in how your child feels. If there's no difference, try cutting out some of the wheat products. Let your pediatrician know what you're doing and ask to have a discussion of the results.

Fill out one diary sheet each day for a minimum of two weeks. Be sure to include snacks and beverages. In the description column, record the symptoms or reaction, whether your child was constipated or had diarrhea, and whether or not she had abdominal bloating, burping, or gas. Don't make a big deal out of it for your child. You want to record her normal eating habits. Also, you don't want your child to become self-conscious about what she's eating.

Keep the sleep diary below for a minimum of two weeks during which your child is not traveling or sleeping in a bed other than his own. Bring this record along with the food diary to your pediatrician to help analyze the results and discover which foods your child may be sensitive to and how they may be affecting your child's sleep patterns.

**Sleep Diary Week of** _____

| Sunday | Bedtime: | Hrs Slept: | Bad Dreams:<br>Yes ❑<br>No ❑ | |
| --- | --- | --- | --- | --- |
| **Monday** | Bedtime: | Hrs Slept: | Bad Dreams:<br>Yes ❑<br>No ❑ | |
| **Tuesday** | Bedtime: | Hrs Slept: | Bad Dreams:<br>Yes ❑<br>No ❑ | |
| **Wednesday** | Bedtime: | Hrs Slept: | Bad Dreams:<br>Yes ❑<br>No ❑ | |
| **Thursday** | Bedtime: | Hrs Slept: | Bad Dreams:<br>Yes ❑<br>No ❑ | |
| **Friday** | Bedtime: | Hrs Slept: | Bad Dreams:<br>Yes ❑<br>No ❑ | |
| **Saturday** | Bedtime: | Hrs Slept: | Bad Dreams:<br>Yes ❑<br>No ❑ | |

Because food sensitivities vary with each child, getting them under control requires a more holistic approach than the symptom-specific ones used to treat allergies. Therein lies the problem. Perhaps because of the newly focused attention to and awareness of allergies, the more subtle diagnoses and treatment of children suffering from intolerances often

| | | | |
|---|---|---|---|
| Urinating or Stooling in the night?<br>Yes ❏<br>No ❏ | Gas/Bloating at bedtime?<br>Yes ❏<br>No ❏ | Napping Hours? | Feeling on Awakening<br>Alert ❏<br>Groggy ❏ |
| Urinating or Stooling in the night?<br>Yes ❏<br>No ❏ | Gas/Bloating at bedtime?<br>Yes ❏<br>No ❏ | Napping Hours? | Feeling on Awakening<br>Alert ❏<br>Groggy ❏ |
| Urinating or Stooling in the night?<br>Yes ❏<br>No ❏ | Gas/Bloating at bedtime?<br>Yes ❏<br>No ❏ | Napping Hours? | Feeling on Awakening<br>Alert ❏<br>Groggy ❏ |
| Urinating or Stooling in the night?<br>Yes ❏<br>No ❏ | Gas/Bloating at bedtime?<br>Yes ❏<br>No ❏ | Napping Hours? | Feeling on Awakening<br>Alert ❏<br>Groggy ❏ |
| Urinating or Stooling in the night?<br>Yes ❏<br>No ❏ | Gas/Bloating at bedtime?<br>Yes ❏<br>No ❏ | Napping Hours? | Feeling on Awakening<br>Alert ❏<br>Groggy ❏ |
| Urinating or Stooling in the night?<br>Yes ❏<br>No ❏ | Gas/Bloating at bedtime?<br>Yes ❏<br>No ❏ | Napping Hours? | Feeling on Awakening<br>Alert ❏<br>Groggy ❏ |
| Urinating or Stooling in the night?<br>Yes ❏<br>No ❏ | Gas/Bloating at bedtime?<br>Yes ❏<br>No ❏ | Napping Hours? | Feeling on Awakening<br>Alert ❏<br>Groggy ❏ |

get missed. Some physicians even go so far as to dismiss the concept of intolerance as "alternative quackery." The problem is compounded by the fact that intolerances do not show up on routine and standard allergy tests. It is not surprising, then, that the solution to many children's relentless symptoms remains elusive.

That's often because the physician is looking at one symptom at a time instead of as a symptom complex, as we discussed in Chapter 1, where commonly linked symptoms frequently appear together. Like little Rowan, your child may have a runny nose and a stomachache, or a rash and a cough, or any combination of respiratory, skin, and gastrointestinal problems. Children with this symptom complex have a heightened response to various food-based triggers, causing them to have symptoms that may seem unrelated, but all actually reflect the same immunological imbalance.

# Questions to Ask Your Child's Doctor

- Should my child be tested for allergies?

- When can I introduce my child to potentially allergenic foods (like peanuts)?

- What should I do if my child gets hives?

- What do I do if the allergy test is negative but I can tell certain foods still upset him, like milk?

- When can I reintroduce foods that seem to make his stomach upset?

# Chapter 4 Take-Home Points

- True allergic reactions cause the body's immune system to develop antibodies against what it perceives to be a foreign invader. The immune system responds by creating specific antibodies called immunoglobulin E, or IgE. Every time you eat this food again, the body sends out IgE antibodies and other chemicals, which can cause a broad variety of inflammatory reactions.

- Allergies are measurable in the blood.

- The eight foods that cause 90 percent of allergic reactions are milk, eggs, peanuts, fish, shellfish, soy, wheat, and tree nuts (like cashews, walnuts, pecans, and almonds).

- If you think your child is allergic to a specific food, visit your pediatrician and take along a food history.

- An intolerance is different from an allergy in that it does not cause your body to generate antibodies against a food. It is caused by a problem in the way the body *processes* a particular food or food additive.

- If your child is suffering from one or more of the symptoms of food intolerance, it's a good idea to keep a food and sleep diary, an organized inventory of what foods and beverages your child is ingesting every day and how these foods are affecting his or her sleep patterns.

As you will find out from the "Let's Get Specific" chapters in Part II of this book, you can identify the sources of your child's imbalances and correct the problem with some very simple and sensible solutions. In fact, if your child is suffering from food intolerances, there are a number of treatment options to help him feel better, be less irritable, and have more energy and concentration. With the right information and some simple planning, symptoms can be managed, controlled, or even eradicated.

# PART II

# NUTRITION AND
# THE IMMUNE SYSTEM

Now that you know how the inclusive category of "food" influences the way your child's body works, it's time to get specific. In this section of the book you'll learn about specific foods and food groups, and why so many of them are so good for us—and so bad for us when they're over-consumed. You'll learn about the pros and cons of wheat, dairy, proteins, and fats. You'll be introduced to probiotics, the friendly bacteria that form a natural defense barrier against harmful bacteria and toxins, which we all need for healthy digestive and immune system function. And you'll discover some supplements you may want to use to bolster your children's good health.

Why do you need to know about these specific foods? So that you as a parent can make the best possible choices for your family. We want to encourage you to broaden your horizons when it comes to food. Try something new. Take a look at what your kids are eating. Are they eating foods that are full of empty calories (soft drinks, energy bars, chips, fat-filled foods)? Are they eating too much of particular foods, like wheat or dairy, and suffering the consequences? You'll be amazed when you find out what kinds of ingredients are added to the foods we feed our children every day. You will not only discover what's wrong with the way we eat in the modern world, you'll discover a whole new way of eating based on human paleological history.

Once you understand how different foods work in your body, you'll begin to look at food in a different way. You'll want to make changes for yourself and for your family. You'll begin to be passionate about providing your family with a rich and complex diet. We understand that getting your kid from eating macaroni and cheese at every meal to a rich and complex diet may seem impossible, but we assure you, small steps will do it.

Here in America, we have a very limited food palate. Help your kids get interested in foods from other cultures, other parts of the world. It used to be, you'd have to shop far and wide to find anything other than a "meat and potatoes" menu. Now virtually every supermarket offers a huge variety of organic and ethnic foods. Take your kids food shopping with you and walk them through the vegetable aisle, pointing out foods they may not see every day. Let them know that there are exciting options to be found in the fruit section. Do they know what a papaya tastes like? A mango? A kiwi? Have they ever seen a live lobster? Let them marvel at all the different colors and kinds of fish for sale. Let them choose one new food to try, and then let them help cook it. Take them on an adventure through the grocery store.

Of course, they won't like everything they try. But surely they will find something to like, and then you can add it to your family's food repertoire, one bite at a time.

# Chapter 5

# Let's Get Specific: Carbohydrates

If you're a parent, you know that your child lives on carbohydrates: french fries, pizza, cookies, bread, macaroni and cheese. They will always choose the carb over any other food. They will reach for the noodle, not the broccoli. You know it's not healthy, but you think, well, they have to eat *something*. You may be wondering how you can get your kids to eat what's good for them. Maybe you believe that you can keep your child from becoming obese by feeding him a low-carb diet, cutting way down on bread, pasta, and potatoes. But not all carbs are bad for you, and eliminating one entire food group is not the way to go, especially for growing children and young adults. After all, it's one thing to make radical food decisions for you and other adults in your household, but quite another thing where children are concerned.

Science tells us that children are not just smaller adults; their bodies and minds, still developing and growing, have different needs than ours do. In order to facilitate this healthy growth, they need to consume a wide range of healthy carbohydrates. This chapter will explain exactly what carbohydrates are, what they do and do not do for your body, and what types of carbs are best for your family's health.

> Our current ways of eating are unfamiliar to our genes, and are causing malfunctions at every level of our health.

## The Evolution of Carbohydrates

Much of what we talked about in previous chapters—the earaches, the tummy aches, the respiratory problems, the cognitive difficulties—stem from the modern American diet's reliance on grain-based starches and carbohydrates. It's the foods we're eating, in the quantities and forms we're eating them, that are making our children sick.

Carbohydrates were not meant to be part of candy bars, frozen foods, chips, or any other foods that were invented by modern man. The carbs our ancestors consumed were eaten in their natural state—fruit directly from the trees, berries from bushes, nuts and seeds most likely found on the ground. Obviously, we have evolved since ancient times. Contrary to popular opinion (and wishful thinking), however, we have not evolved to be able to tolerate the huge volumes of sugar and carbohydrates that are part of the modern American diet. According to modern science, the human genome has changed little in the past 40,000 years. In fact, 99.9 percent of our genes date much farther back than 40,000 years, and were therefore formed way before the development of agriculture.

What does this mean? The implication is that our current ways of eating are unfamiliar to our genes and are causing malfunctions at every level of our health. The disparity between what we are evolved to eat and what we are currently eating is making us older, fatter, and sicker than we should be. And it's causing our kids to suffer from the multiple symptoms described in earlier chapters.

Think about it: Human beings are the only primates that are high grain consumers. No other primate has access to the volume or variety of grains that we do. It is the development of agriculture that made the difference, and although we enjoy the benefits of that discovery, we also suffer its consequences.

Agriculture brought the cultivation of plant crops and cereal grains. Although cereal grains are the foundation of modern dietary guidelines worldwide, they have been central to the human diet for only a moment in our evolution. And now we are moving in leaps and bounds to hypermodify foods. Our bodies—and in particular, children's little bodies—have had no time at all to adapt to these man-made super-high-energy foods devoid of many if not all of the phytochemicals that are healthiest for growth and development. When we mix modern technologies of food processing with the marvels of present-day marketing tactics, we are creating kids who only want the foods they see on TV—foods that are packed with sugar and damaging fats, laced with hormone-disrupting chemicals, and bloated with calories!

........................................................................

### Phyto What?

Phytochemicals, also known as phytonutrients, are health-protecting compounds found in fruits, vegetables, and other plants. There are thousands of phytochemicals found in the plant world. While plants produce these chemicals to protect themselves, scientists have shown that they can also protect humans against diseases. Some of the best-known phytochemicals are lycopene in tomatoes, isoflavones in soy, and flavonoids in fruits.

........................................................................

Our ancestors did not have the kinds of food choices we have available to us today. They didn't have breads, pastas, grains, and sugar-laden desserts. If they craved sweets, it was because they needed the vitamin C that fruits (such as berries, mangoes, papaya, bananas, and so on) provided. Whatever they consumed worked efficiently with their bodies' own chemistry.

The problem with today's modern diet is that much of it—the huge amounts of sugar and processed carbohydrates—does not react well with our bodies' chemistry, and, in fact, wreaks havoc with our health and well-being. That's because these substances adversely affect those chemicals in our bodies, known as hormones, that are our bodies' biological messengers. They tell our organs, cells, and tissues what to do and when. The hormonal (or endocrine) system is one of the body's great communications networks. Hormones are involved in just about every biological process: immune function, reproduction, growth, even controlling other hormones. And they work in extremely small concentrations, which is why it is so easy for even minute doses of harmful substances to disrupt their functioning efficiency and cause miscommunication, which can eventually lead to the disease and destruction of our bodies' cells.

## Carb Facts

What are carbohydrates anyway? They are mainly sugars and starches and are one of the three principal types of nutrients used as energy sources by the body (the other two are proteins and fats, which will be detailed in later chapters). Carbohydrates are made up of chains of sugar molecules. Even carbs that don't seem to be sugary—like bread, bagels, and pasta—are made up of sugar molecules.

---

### From Simple to Complex

Carbohydrates are usually categorized in two ways: simple and complex. You could also think of them as sugars and starches. Simple carbs are sugar molecules that are quickly and easily digested and absorbed through the intestines. Some foods with simple carbs are sugar, corn syrup, maple syrup, honey, and most fruit. Complex carbohydrates, which are found in starchy foods like whole grains, potatoes, and vegetables, are made up of simple sugar molecules linked together.

---

The body uses carbohydrates primarily for energy. In fact, carbs supply every cell in your body with the energy they need. Here's some basic science for you:

You eat a carbohydrate.

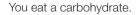

The body turns the carb into glucose (sugar).

The body uses as much glucose as it needs for immediate fuel.

Cells can use only so much glucose at one time.
The unused glucose is converted to glycogen
and stored in your liver and muscle cells.
If there's still more glycogen left over, it is turned to fat.

If you need a quick spurt of energy for a sport, activity, or emergency, the body will release stores of glycogen. If you're engaged in a longer activity, like taking a hike or playing in a nine-inning softball game, the body turns to fat for fuel.

Some carbs also provide us with fiber, important to the digestive process because it gets food to move more quickly through the large intestine, reducing the risk of digestive disorders (including constipation, commonly caused in children by low fiber intake). Fiber also helps us feel full after a meal, which can help prevent kids from overeating and reduce their tendencies to clamor for snacks before bedtime.

Carbohydrates rich in fiber include green leafy vegetables such as spinach, watercress, lettuces (including mesclun), and a wide variety of sprouts. Add in vegetables like tomatoes, carrots, peapods, asparagus, zucchini, peppers, radishes, and cucumbers; and cooked cruciferous vegetables such as broccoli, kale, cauliflower, cabbage, and brussels sprouts, and your family's fiber intake will be more than adequate.

Okay, so maybe your kids won't eat brussels sprouts. They will most likely eat seeds, nuts, and fruits—foods that figured prominently in the ancestral diet.

- Try to include fruits that are rich in natural antioxidants and vitamin C. Antioxidants are chemical substances that help protect against cell damage from free radicals. Free radicals are nasty molecular terrorists that are linked to everything from illness to aging to heart disease to genetic changes that can trigger cancer. It's only in the past few decades that we've begun to understand how damaging free radicals can be and how important it is to have plenty of antioxidants in our bodies to neutralize them. Blueberries and strawberries, for instance, are rich in antioxidants. Blueberries have been shown to improve both coordination and short-term memory, according to a United States Department of Agriculture study. Besides being potent antioxidants, blueberries also have anti-inflammatory and blood-thinning effects.

- Apples are rich in naturally occurring antioxidants known as phenolics and flavonoids.

- All fruits and vegetables are healthy—fresh, frozen, canned, or dried (when choosing canned fruit, look for labels that say, "no sugar added"). They can be eaten raw, steamed, roasted, boiled, microwaved, or stir-fried. Strive to have a variety of different types of fruits and vegetables from all the different color groups (yellow, green, and red).

Fiber-rich fruits and vegetables are packed with phytochemicals that are essential to protect the body's immune system, especially the developing immune system of a child. They were part of our ancestral diet, as opposed to the highly processed and refined foods we are now feeding our children, which tend to be calorically dense, high in fat and salt, and much higher in sugar than most children need to consume in order to be well and healthy.

So you can see how important the right carbohydrates are to our well-being. In fact, the United States government's official food pyramid tells you to base your diet on grains and carbohydrates. We suggest that you take a lesson from your ancestors, turn that notion around, and feed your children (and yourself) a diet based on fiber-rich fruits and vegetables and lean proteins, with moderate servings of whole grains. The rest of this chapter will explain why we feel that way.

## GOOD CARBS, BAD CARBS, AND THE GLYCEMIC INDEX

In the 1980s, a group of scientists decided there needed to be an easy way to identify which carbs were good for you and which were not so good. They developed what they called the glycemic index (GI), designed to measure how rapidly a carbohydrate is absorbed into your bloodstream and its potential impact on insulin secretion. Each carbohydrate is assigned a number that reflects the rate at which it causes glucose (sugar) levels in the blood to rise. The higher the number, the faster the carb converts to glucose in the blood. The goal is to keep that number low. If you eat a meal loaded with high-GI carbs, you cause insulin levels to soar (and then drop rapidly). The higher a food's glycemic value, the faster it enters the bloodstream. When that happens, the pancreas responds by secreting insulin. While that does bring blood sugar levels down, it also tells the body to store fat and keep it stored. Over time this will not only make you fat, it will also keep you and your children fat. In contrast, a meal with low-GI carbs raises blood sugar slowly and steadily.

Foods on the glycemic index are scored on a scale of 0 to 100, 100 being the absolute value of pure glucose (sugar). The lower the glycemic value of a food, the better. The higher the value, the closer it gets to pure sugar in your blood (very bad).

Here is a small sampling of some carbs and their glycemic values:

| Food | Glycemic Score |
| --- | --- |
| Peas (split, dried, yellow, green) | 22 |
| Barley | 25 |
| Red kidney beans | 27 |
| Black beans | 30 |
| Lentils | 30 |
| Chickpeas | 33 |
| Oats | 49 |
| Yam | 51 |
| Sweet potato | 54 |
| Taro root | 54 |
| Kasha | 54 |
| Maize, corn | 55 |
| Brown rice | 55 |
| Basmati rice | 58 |
| Couscous | 65 |

> ## We Can't Live by Numbers Alone
>
> The glycemic index is a guide, not a rulebook, and here's why: Numbers can be deceiving. Carrots and watermelon, for instance, both have very high GI values, but they also have a lot of fiber and are full of phytonutrients. If you went simply by the numbers, you might skip a healthy and delicious food. The absorption of carbohydrates can be slowed down if you also ingest fat (such as fish oil, olive oil, sesame oil, or butter) along with them. For instance, if you eat fish (which obviously contains fish oil) with rice on the side, the oil modifies the glycemic impact of the rice on your bloodstream, or the rate of its conversion and absorption into blood sugar.

## BEWARE OVERCONSUMPTION OF SUGAR AND CARBOHYDRATES

We all want our children to grow up to be healthy, happy adults. That is why it's so important to set them on the right nutritional path from the very beginning. The damage that an imbalance or lack of proper nutrients can cause affects your child long after he or she is grown. After years of eating breads, pastas, noodles, cakes, cookies, pizzas, muffins, cereals, and refined sugars, the tissue in our bodies becomes rigid and pigmented (producing age spots) with deposits of tissue-stiffening

**Sugar-driven damage accumulates as we age and accelerates the deterioration of *all* our functions and capabilities.**

compounds called Advanced Glycation End Products, or AGEs. The overconsumption of sugar and carbohydrates, in all their forms, produces these stiff sugar protein bonds that accumulate in our bodies as we get older. These bonds are a result of sugar "gluing" itself to our collagen, veins, arteries, ligaments, bones, brains—you name it, producing a constellation of changes, including stiff joints, hardened arteries, failing organs, and enfeebled muscles. Sugar will combine with almost anything. It's extremely sticky—just think of sugar drying on your fingers. Sugar-driven damage accumulates as we age and accelerates the deterioration of all our functions and capabilities.

Here are some facts about sugar:

- Sugar consumption in 1821 was 10 pounds per person per year. Currently it's about 156 pounds per person per year (noncaloric sweeteners add another 50 pounds per person per year).

- In the American diet, the major source of added sugar—not including naturally occurring sugars, like the fructose in fruit—is soft drinks. They account for 33 percent of all added sugars consumed. Another 26 percent of added sugars comes from a variety of prepared foods like ketchup, canned vegetables and fruits, and peanut butter.

- Pepsi contains 1.2 teaspoons of sugar per ounce of soda. Most cans contain 12 ounces, for a whopping 14.4 teaspoons of sugar per can.

- Quaker Instant Oatmeal in cinnamon or spice flavors packs 4.3 teaspoons of sugar per ounce.

- Heinz Custard Pudding (baby food) contains 4 teaspoons of sugar. Is that really necessary? In fact, according to a May 2009 survey conducted by the Children's Food Campaign in England, some brands of baby food contain as much sugar and saturated fats as cookies and cheeseburgers. The group said some baby foods billed as being healthy are worse than junk food in terms of sugar, salt, and trans fats, which is a leading cause of deadly heart disease.

- Ounce-per-ounce, most breakfast cereals (including Honeycomb, Froot Loops, and Cocoa Puffs) contain more sugar than a soft drink.

## A Doughnut or a Bowl of Cereal?

Most parents would not consider feeding their children doughnuts for breakfast. It's pretty obvious that a doughnut or similar pastry contains a lot of sugar. But a 2008 analysis by *Consumer Reports* found that eleven popular cereals contain at least 40 percent sugar per serving. That's as much sugar per serving as you get in a glazed doughnut from Dunkin' Donuts. Two cereals—Post Golden Crisp and Kellogg's Honey Smacks—contain more than 50 percent sugar by weight. And every parent knows that when children pour their own bowls of cereal, they're getting more than one serving's worth (in fact, according to the report, they're pouring at least 50 percent more than the suggested serving). The four brands that were deemed "very good" were Cheerios, Kix, Life, and Honey Nut Cheerios. Other recommendations include Kashi 7 Whole Grain Honey Puffs, Kashi Mighty Bites, and Kellogg's All-Bran Yogurt Bites.

Unfortunately, sugar isn't the only food source that is causing problems for today's children. Many of the problems outlined in this book are caused by grains, specifically, corn and wheat.

## CHILDREN OF THE CORN

As any kid will tell you, one of the best things about summer is sweet yellow corn on the cob. And you might think that by serving corn you're giving your child a good vegetable option. You might be surprised to learn, however, that corn is not a vegetable at all—it's a grain. It's still a great treat for a summer Sunday barbeque. But since the 1970s something has happened to our delicious ear of corn, something that's helped to turn our children into heavier, more disease-prone toddlers, teens, and young adults. In fact, there are two distinct ways that this sweet summer treat has turned into a danger for our society's future.

First, let's talk about high-fructose corn syrup (HFCS). High-fructose corn syrup is a common sweetener and preservative, made by changing the sugar (glucose) in cornstarch to fructose—another form of sugar. The end product is a combination of fructose and glucose that extends the shelf life of processed foods and is cheaper than sugar. You can see how that combination would make it so popular amongst food manufacturers. HFCS is the primary sweetener used in the United States right now. And it is found in an astounding array of foods: candy, beverages, cereals, breads, cookies, crackers, yogurt, ice cream, salad dressing, steak sauce, pancake syrup, pasta sauce, ketchup, canned soups, fruit juice, soft drinks, and even cough syrup.

So what's the problem? Several studies have shown that unlike glucose, fructose is readily converted to fat by the liver, contributing to fat deposits in the liver (which we don't want) and leading to an excessive concentration of fats and lipoproteins (protein compounds that carry fats and fat-like substances, such as cholesterol, in the blood) in the body. This can eventually lead to plaque buildup in the blood vessels. It can also lead to gout, kidney stones, obesity, and Type 2 diabetes.

All these sound like very adult problems—but they are beginning to develop at alarming rates in the adolescent and young adult populations. HFCS does not contain any vitamins, minerals, or phytochemicals— just calories. So in the long run, the only benefit of all this high-fructose corn syrup is for the food industry, not you or your children.

### Give Up Fructose? No Way!

We would never suggest that you eliminate fructose from your child's diet. After all, fructose is found in fruits, and kids should have all the phytonutrients they provide. It's the overconsumption of fructose that is the problem, and high-fructose corn syrup is everywhere. What's a concerned parent to do? Read the label. If HFCS (or just fructose) is one of the first ingredients listed, make

> another choice. If you want to give your child a treat every once
> in a while, do so. But try to find ways to cut down. If you want to
> give your child fruit juice, for example, which often contains HFCS,
> dilute it with sparkling water. It tastes just as sweet but cuts the
> fructose in half.

### Corn, Cows, and Kids

There is another issue concerning corn and your kids' health, and it has to do with cows (and chickens, too). A November 2008 study in the Proceedings of the National Academy of Sciences looked at the beef and chicken served at fast food chains including McDonald's, Burger King, and Wendy's. They found that virtually all the meat served at these restaurants came from animals that have been fed corn.

Corn itself is not inherently unhealthy. That ear (or two) consumed at dinner won't harm your children's health. The problem is that corn has entered every aspect of the food chain. Take beef, for instance. Kids love hamburgers, don't they? What they don't know is that virtually all the burgers in their Happy Meals comes from cattle that are fed primarily corn, corn husks, and corn stalks. But cows are not designed to live on corn. Cows are designed to live on grasses. Raising a cow to full weight and sale capacity on grass requires on enormous amount of time, a lot more than the market cycle permits. One of the quickest ways to fatten a cow is to feed it primarily corn.

So? So beef that comes from corn-fed cattle is high in saturated fats, which is known to clog arteries. And corn-fed beef is lower in healthy substances like omega-3 fatty acids, which we know are heart-healthy.

And, since cows were not designed to eat corn, the grain tends to mess with their digestive systems. These cows die younger if they're just fed corn, so they're given antibiotics to keep them from getting sick. Those antibiotics—not to mention the pesticides that are sprayed on the corn—are transferred to you and your child when you eat the meat.

## What's the Alternative?

Go organic if you can. We realize that organic beef and chicken can be expensive. But organic is not as elitist as it used to be, and prices are going down in some areas. Not too long ago, you could only find organic meats at Whole Foods and local health food stores. These days, however, more large chain supermarkets (like Wal-Mart and Kroger's, for example) carry organic foods. There are also many food co-ops around that offer lower prices. It's worth your child's health to do a little shopping around to find the best you can afford. And if your kid wants fast food and likes Mexican, you might want to try a once-in-a-while trip to Chipotle. This chain lets you build your own burrito, taco, or salad with fresh ingredients, organic hormone- and antibiotic-free meats, and produce sourced from local suppliers.

Not everything you buy needs to be organic, however. Here are some simple rules for when to buy organic and when it's not necessary:

- **Buy organic when the skin is thin.** Fruits and vegetables with thin skins that are difficult to remove or that you usually eat should be organic. They do not have the same type of barrier against pesticides that thick-skinned fruits and veggies have.

- **Thin-skinned examples** include apples, strawberries, peaches, raspberries, blueberries, blackberries, grapes, pears, cherries, nectarines, celery, potatoes, and carrots.

- **Thick-skinned examples** include avocados, bananas, eggplants, corn, kiwi, papaya, mangoes, squash, oranges, and grapefruit.

- **Leafy greens should be organic.** Anything that is leafy like lettuce should be organic because you can't completely wash every leaf. Vegetables that should be organic include all types of lettuce, kale, spinach, collard greens, mustard greens, and Swiss chard. Vegetables that don't need to be organic include broccoli, cabbage, asparagus, cauliflower, and sweet potatoes.

- **Dairy should be organic.** This industry uses a lot of hormones and antibiotics, so buy organic milk, cheese, and yogurt whenever possible. Also, organic milk has higher levels of omega-3 fatty acids (see Chapter 7), which is good for your health.

- **Meat and poultry should be organic.** The same warning about hormones and antibiotics applies here as well.

- **Fish and seafood do not need to be organic.** Fish live in the ocean and (hopefully) do not encounter as many pesticides and toxins as other foods.

## HOW TO KEEP A PICKY CHILD HEALTHY

There are no tricks to getting kids to eat. You need to know that kids don't starve themselves. If you're giving them healthy food and they don't eat it right away, don't push them. Eventually they will eat it because they're hungry. Just keep offering them the same healthy choices and before you know it, they will get hungry enough to put it in their mouths.

What frequently happens is that you make a healthy meal and your child won't eat it. Then the power play begins. Children are smart. They know that pitching a fit will usually get them what they want. Even parents who send their kids away from the table if they won't eat end up giving in later in the day when the child cries and says, "I'm hungry." If that happens, offer your child the same healthy food he or she rejected earlier.

Food is not a punishment or a reward. It doesn't help to yell and scream, "If you don't eat this broccoli now, you will not have dinner and you will eat it cold for breakfast." Who would behave after that kind of threat? And if you say, "If you eat your broccoli now you can have ice cream for dessert," they will never learn to appreciate vegetables—they'll eat a bite or two just to collect the goodie at the end of the meal.

And don't forget that you are the model for eating healthy food. The more you have the right food around and the more you give them healthy choices, the more likely it is that they will learn the right way to eat.

Here are some adjustments you can make to simple meals so that you know your child is getting as many nutrients as possible:

- **Pasta:** Many picky eaters rely solely on pasta for dinner and/or lunch. Some with butter, some with cheese, and some with sauce. You can get a little more nutrition in them by substituting whole wheat pasta for regular pasta, thereby introducing some whole grains into their diet. Whole grains are said to reduce the risk of heart disease, cancer, and diabetes, and are full of vitamins and minerals.

- **Snacks:** Whole-rye crackers with some cream cheese can be a healthy snack, so can popping your own plain popcorn. Keep some dried fruit on hand for when you go out.

- **Drinks:** Limit high-calorie drinks, which fill kids up before mealtimes. Make good fruit juice choices. Pick juices with the least amount of sugar. If your child doesn't like dairy foods, buy one of their favorite fruit juices with calcium added to it. For example, Ocean Spray has a great Cranberry Juice Cocktail with calcium.

- **Fruit:** If your child isn't a big fruit eater, try making her a smoothie! You can use tofu to add protein without changing the taste and texture, as well as some ground flaxseed for fiber and omega-3 oil for fat. Add fortified fruit juice, yogurt, or frozen yogurt if you want to add some calcium.

# Questions to Ask Your Child's Doctor

- My child eats primarily carbohydrates. Of all the options, which ones would you recommend for daily consumption?

- We both agree that my child is overweight. Some people say that I should stop giving her carbs. Do you think that is the way to go? Is it safe to try for a while?

- My son's teachers tell me he is very low-energy in school. Do you think it's because he only eats pasta, or is there something else that might be causing it?

- Should he be tested for anemia before I assume it's his carbohydrate-laden diet that is causing his fatigue?

- My child is so picky that if I don't serve her pasta she will skip dinner altogether. Is she growing well? Can I stop worrying and teach her to eat the protein or be hungry?

- I am concerned about school lunches. It seems like the menu consists of nothing but spaghetti or some other form of pasta. Can you help me write a letter to the principal?

# Chapter 5 Take-Home Points

- Don't stop feeding your children carbohydrates. Breads, potatoes, rice, and pasta should remain a part of your family's diet. These foods can be prepared in very healthy and interesting ways and provide important nutrients for growing children and teens. Keep in mind that nutrition is a key driver of performance in school and that proper nutrition comes from a balanced diet.

- We suggest a diet that's rich in multiple sources of starches and carbohydrates, including rice, quinoa, millet, some oats, and corn on the cob, with additional starches coming from beans, legumes, root vegetables, yams, and surface vegetables (squashes and pumpkins) of all kinds.

- Watch portion sizes, especially when eating at restaurants. Portion sizes continue to creep upward, and research shows that Americans have an amazing ability to finish whatever is put on their plates. For example, some restaurants serve 6 cups of pasta in a regular order. One to 2 cups should suffice for dinner. Don't let restaurants decide how many calories or carbs you want or need. You be the judge.

- Serve whole grain/high-fiber breads and cereals rather than refined grain products. Look for "whole grain" as the first ingredient on the food label and make at least half your grain servings whole grain. The American Heart Association's recommended grain intake ranges from 2 ounces per day for a one-year-old to 7 ounces per day for a fourteen- to eighteen-year-old boy.

- Serve a variety of fruits and vegetables daily, while limiting juice intake. Each meal should contain at least one fruit or vegetable. Children's recommended fruit intake ranges from 1 cup per day, between ages one and three, to 2 cups a day for fourteen- to eighteen-year-old boys. Recommended vegetable intake ranges

**79**

from three-fourths of a cup a day at age one to 3 cups for a fourteen- to eighteen-year-old boy.

- Be sure to serve carbohydrates that are rich in fiber, including green leafy vegetables such as spinach, watercress, lettuces (including mesclun), and a wide variety of sprouts. Add in vegetables like tomatoes, carrots, peapods, asparagus, zucchini, peppers, radishes, and cucumbers; and cooked cruciferous vegetables such as broccoli, kale, cauliflower, and cabbage. And don't forget seeds, nuts, and fruits.

- Read all food labels. Try to avoid foods that have high-fructose corn syrup (or any other form of fructose) as one of the first ingredients listed.

There is one more topic regarding carbohydrates that must be covered because it is so prevalent—and causing so many problems—in the modern American diet today. That is why the next chapter is solely devoted to the subject of wheat.

# Chapter 6

# Let's Get Specific: Wheat

There's been a lot of talk about wheat lately—most of it confusing. Are we supposed to eat wheat or not? Are we supposed to eat whole wheat or no wheat? And if there are so many questions about adults eating wheat, who's asking about the kids? Not to mention the fact that there's wheat in so many things we eat, from breakfast and snacks right through to dinner and on to dessert. Why does it cause so many problems? And do we even know what those problems are?

Like everything else we talk about in this book, wheat has its good points and its bad points. But be assured that although there are a variety of problems caused by the *overconsumption* of wheat, you do not have to send your kids to Wheat Eaters Anonymous or assume that even one bite of a cookie or slice of pizza means they are doomed to disease.

Wheat is, in fact, the most important cereal crop in the world. It is deeply embedded in the food culture of North America and many other regions of the world. Bread, pasta, pizza, bagels, cereal, crackers, cakes, and muffins are just the start of a long list of foods made with wheat.

Problems arise because, as we learned in the last chapter, humans have not evolved to consume so many grains, whether they're whole wheat or refined grain products. High grain consumption is a relatively new addition to the human diet, beginning with the agricultural age approximately 12,000 years ago. It wasn't until recently (in terms of human history) that human beings gave up much of the variety they used to have in their diets and became heavily reliant on a small subset of carbohydrates. We now know that corn is one carb in that subset. The other is wheat.

Whole wheat (in its original form) is a good source of dietary fiber, manganese, and magnesium. And studies have shown that whole wheat can help lower the risk of type 2 diabetes, heart disease, chronic inflammation, gallstones, and breast cancer.

However, the fiber and most of the other nutrients in wheat come from its hard outer layer, called *bran,* and the *germ,* the inner part of a wheat kernel, both of which are removed when the grain is milled to produce white flour (products that are made from whole wheat include the bran and the germ).

Refined grains and the foods made from them (e.g., white breads, cookies, pastries, pasta, and rice) are now being linked not only to weight gain but to increased risk of insulin resistance (the precursor of type 2 diabetes) and metabolic syndrome (a strong predictor of both type 2 diabetes and cardiovascular disease). Most of the grains that are consumed (and overconsumed) today deliver very high amounts of concentrated energy calories but don't necessarily deliver many health benefits. For instance, we know that broccoli offers certain kinds of phytochemicals that fight cancer and other disease. There don't seem to be too many destructive side effects of overconsuming broccoli. Unfortunately, that can't be said for the high consumption of grains made from refined wheat.

## PROBLEM #1: GLUTEN

Why does eating so much wheat cause us problems? There are actually several reasons, the first of which is gluten, a macro-molecule that's part of the whole wheat seed. Gluten appears to produce multiple detrimental effects within the immune system, especially within a child's immune system and a child's bowel. A little gluten won't harm most people. But most people—especially most children—ingest more than a little gluten every day.

Most of us aren't even aware of how much wheat we eat in a day, much less how much our kids eat. But follow a kid around for a day, and you might be surprised at how quickly the wheat intake adds up. Let's take little Zach, for instance. Zach wakes up and has a bowl of cereal for breakfast. Since he's poured it himself, he's probably having at least two servings in his bowl. Later on it's getting toward noon but lunch is not ready yet, so Zach reaches for a pretzel stick (or two) to tide him over. At lunch, he has a peanut butter and jelly sandwich on two slices of white bread. Then at a playdate with his best friend he has a crunchy granola bar and a glass of milk. And finally, he has a bowl of macaroni and cheese (because he's in his "mac 'n cheese" phase and won't eat anything else) for dinner. It's a typical day for an active four-year-old. Let's review: wheat for breakfast, wheat for snack, wheat for lunch, a late-day wheat snack, and wheat for dinner. Gluten overload, anyone?

But it gets worse. Gluten is also used as a thickener or stabilizing agent in products like ice cream, canned soup, pie fillings, salad dressings, ketchup, and even Play-Doh (the Hasbro Web site for Play-Doh contains this warning: "Children who are allergic to wheat gluten may have an allergic reaction to this product").

---

### A General Rule of Thumb

Because the Food and Drug Administration has classified gluten as GRAS (generally recognized as safe), it is not necessarily listed on food labels. However, if you find any of the following words on food labels, it usually means that a grain containing gluten has been used:

- stabilizer

- modified food starch (prominent in candy)

- monosodium glutamate (MSG)

- flavoring

- emulsifier

- hydrolyzed vegetable protein

- plant protein

- caramel coloring

If you're looking for an easy way to determine if gluten is in the food you're considering purchasing, here's a general rule of thumb to follow: If there are more than five ingredients listed, you can be pretty sure one of them is going to be gluten (probably disguised as one of the terms listed above).

---

**This frequent, chronic exposure for a body that doesn't have the capability to digest this much gluten causes all sorts of problems and disorders, from ear infections and stomachaches, to the common problems of gas and bloating, constipation, lethargy, and so on.**

This frequent, chronic exposure for a body that doesn't have the capability to digest this much gluten causes all sorts of problems and disorders, from ear infections and stomachaches, to the common problems of gas and bloating, constipation, lethargy, and so on. In some children there is a possible link between high grain-based diets and ADD and ADHD, irritable bowel syndrome, and candida overgrowth (candida is a form of yeast normally found in the body at low levels), commonly seen in children who ingest too much gluten and/or sugar.

The good news is that there are an increasing number of gluten-free products on the market, including gluten-free breads and pastas (see "Appendix A: Resource Guide"). But it's important to note that "wheat free" doesn't necessarily mean gluten free. The product may still contain rye, barley, or spelt ingredients that contain gluten.

## PROBLEM #2: LECTIN

There is another compound in wheat that also causes problems. It's called *lectin,* and it is a tiny molecule that selectively causes blood and other body tissues to stick together. Actually, all foods contain lectins, but while they are benign in some foods, they are toxic in others. Foods with high concentrations of lectins, such as beans, cereal grains, seeds, and nuts, may be harmful if consumed in excess. This means that in some foods (particularly wheat, dairy—especially when cows have been grain-fed—and legumes), lectins are more likely to cause sensitivities and/or allergies.

Wheat probably has the highest concentration of lectin of all foods. As it moves through the colon, the lectin works as a kind of chemical key that opens up pathways into cells. As a result, it can cause openings through the bowel walls directly into the general body cavity and can contribute to inflammation, food sensitivities, intolerances, and allergies. When wheat and wheat products are overconsumed on a regular basis, the bowel itself can begin to develop mild inflammation. In an extreme example you have celiac disease, where there's complete destruction of the bowel wall. But in children with sensitivities, tiny tears can begin to show up in the bowel wall and can cause inflammation throughout the body. High lectin/gluten consumption in children has also been associated with asthma, low blood sugar, fatigue, different forms of pain such as fibromyalgia, autoimmune diseases, ADD, ADHD, poor adrenal function, obesity, and higher susceptibility to viruses and infections.

> In some foods (particularly wheat, dairy—especially when cows have been grain-fed—and legumes), lectins are more likely to cause sensitivities and/or allergies.

Unlike gluten, there are no lectin-free foods. The only way to combat lectin's harmful effect is to reduce the overload. That's where Goldilocks comes in.

### The Goldilocks Principle

We all know the story of *Goldilocks and the Three Bears*. She stumbles into the bears' house, in which there is three of everything. She tries three bowls of porridge, sits in three chairs, and lies down in three beds. In each instance, she eventually finds the one that is "just right" for her. That's the way you should approach the subject of wheat.

**A small minority of children can have no wheat at all.** These kids are truly allergic to wheat and probably have what is known as celiac disease, a digestive disorder that interferes with the absorption of nutrients from food. Some common symptoms of celiac disease are diarrhea, decreased appetite, stomachache and bloating, poor growth, and weight loss. Many kids are diagnosed with it when they're between six months and two years old, which is when foods with gluten are first introduced into their diets. This is a serious disease that requires strict adherence to a gluten-free diet.

**Some children will have no reaction whatsoever to wheat** and can eat as much as they like (not that we're advocating for anyone to go overboard where wheat is concerned).

**Many children have wheat sensitivities.** As we explained in Chapter 4, this is not a full-blown allergy. It does not require complete elimination of wheat from the diet. The majority of these children can have moderate amounts of wheat and wheat products. But it does take careful monitoring.

Say for example that your child is going to a birthday party on Saturday. There's going to be cake, for sure. And the hostess is serving pizza. You have a couple of options:

1. You can forbid your child from having the cake and/or the pizza.

2. You teach your child to eat the cheese and tomato off the pizza and leave the crust.

3. You let your child enjoy the cake, the pizza, and the rest of the party.

Option 1 is not a good idea. You don't want your child to feel different, or like she's a little freak, or as if she's being punished. You don't want to instill the idea that food is the enemy.

Option 2 is better, if your child doesn't mind and can be trusted to do this even if you're not around to supervise.

Option 3 is probably best. Let your kid be a kid. Just be sure that that's his wheat allotment for the day. Don't give him cereal for breakfast, and don't make pasta for dinner. Maybe stay away from wheat the next day as well, or at least limit the wheat intake to one or two servings.

It may take some experimentation, but eventually you'll find what is "just right" for your child.

### It's 10:00 a.m. Do You Know Where Your Wheat Is?

*When Julie, a first-time parent, brought her four-year-old daughter Madison in to see me for the third time with a painful earache, I asked her what Madison had been eating lately. On her two previous visits, I had suggested that Julie modify the amount of wheat in Madison's diet. Since I had given Madison antibiotics twice before, I did not want to give her a third round. In answer to my question, Julie replied, "She's not eating that much wheat."*

*"What does she have for breakfast?" I asked.*

*"Hardly anything," said Julie. "Just a bagel with butter."*

*"A bagel?"*

*"Yes," said Julie, "but it's not a wheat bagel. It's multigrain."*

*She felt a bit foolish when I explained that the operative word here was grain, which usually means wheat. When she substituted a gluten-free cereal for Madison's daily breakfast, the earaches disappeared. This example may be a bit extreme, but it shows the importance of learning to recognize ingredients when they're not exactly spelled out for you.*

*—From Dr. Geary's files*

## PUTTING IT ALL TOGETHER

When you put together what we discussed in the last chapter (high-fructose corn syrup) and what we discussed in this chapter (wheat, gluten, and lectin), you can see why the modern American diet is causing such problems for our children. A hamburger is not just a hamburger anymore. When you eat a hamburger, you're eating essentially saturated, fat-laden, corn-fed protein. The bun contains high-fructose corn syrup, which has been embedded into the wheat, along with gluten and lectin. Pour on the ketchup, which has been thickened with gluten and sweetened with high-fructose corn syrup, and you've got corn and wheat again. This is what's building up sensitivities and intolerances in individuals above and beyond what we would consider a direct food allergy. Without realizing it, we've now moved into these very limited food sources.

> When you eat a hamburger, you're eating essentially saturated, fat-laden, corn-fed protein.

The human body is designed to be omnivorous and to choose from an enormous variety of proteins, vegetables, fruits, seeds, beans, and legumes—foods that actually offer phytochemicals that we are no longer getting when we rely too much on corn and wheat.

### Never Say Never

The fundamental principle of this book is "never say never" unless you're talking about children who have true allergies. If your child is allergic to gluten, don't feed him bread or any food that has gluten in it. Ever. But most children don't have allergies; they have sensitivities. That means moderation. We don't want you to be the food police. We don't want you to have to make feeding your child a full-time job. High-fructose corn syrup and processed, refined wheat products are everywhere. You can't control every bite of food your kid takes every day. And you don't have to. You can, instead, manage what your children eat. You may not be able to eliminate all wheat from your child's diet, but you can limit the number of wheat-based meals and snacks he has in one twenty-four-hour period. If, every once in a while, little ones have too many cookies or pizza or pasta in one day, it's not the end of the world. Tomorrow is another day, and another chance to manage how much wheat they consume.

## TESTING FOR SENSITIVITY

If your child is experiencing the earaches, tummy aches, and/or respiratory problems that are related to the atopic triangle, it may be due to wheat sensitivities. How can you find out? By conducting a Wheat Washout. Eliminate wheat from your child's diet for anywhere from two weeks to a month and measure your child's health and cognitive performance when the time period is up. Has he had any more earaches? Has he stopped complaining about stomachaches? Is he doing better in school? Have you made fewer trips to the pediatrician? Then gradually add small amounts of wheat back in. When the symptoms return, you know you've reached your child's limit.

Here are some grains you can substitute during the Wheat Washout:

- Quinoa

- Gluten-free oats

- Barley

- Brown rice

- Millet

- Rye

- Buckwheat

- Amaranth

## Questions to Ask Your Child's Doctor

- Lately I have read a lot about celiac disease. How do I know if my child might have it?

- If I have my child tested for celiac disease and the results are negative, does that mean he can eat as much wheat as he wants?

- Can you develop wheat intolerance, or are you born with it? My daughter seems to get very bloated when she eats wheat, but only since she turned three.

- What other sources of grain besides wheat do you recommend?

- If my child gets bloated after eating birthday cake or pizza but not after pasta, does that mean he is not wheat intolerant?

- If I remove wheat from his diet for two weeks, is that dangerous to his growth?

# Chapter 6 Take-Home Points

- In most cases, you don't have to completely eliminate wheat from your child's diet. Remember the Goldilocks Principle and find the amount that is just right for your child.

- Health problems arise because we are eating so much of so few grains—mainly corn and wheat. Try to add more variety of gluten-free grains to your family's daily fare.

- Read food labels. Check for words like stabilizer, emulsifier, and hydrolyzed, which indicate the presence of gluten. Recognize that if a product has more than five ingredients, gluten is probably one of them.

- Try a two- to four-week Wheat Washout to see if it makes a difference in your child's health.

Wheat is not the only food that can cause problems for children (and adults). It could be that the chronic upset stomachs and digestive issues your child is facing come from one of the most popular staples of the American diet: milk. In the next chapter, you'll find out you just might want to answer the question "Got milk?" with a resounding "No!"

CHAPTER 7

# Let's Get Specific: Dairy

Growing up in America, we are led to believe that milk, notably cow's milk, is a critical part of a healthy child's diet. We have all seen the advertisements that feature celebrities with a milk mustache, and milk and cookies is as American as apple pie . . . *but do kids really need milk?*

Cow's milk provides your child with three critical ingredients: fat, calcium, and vitamin D. It also provides them with a potential milk-protein allergy, microscopic gastritis, or lactose intolerance. Other sources of fat, calcium, and vitamin D, which will be laid out in this and other chapters, are worth trying, too.

If you're a parent, the most important information you need is the difference between lactose intolerance and a milk allergy. Lactose intolerance is a deficiency in the enzyme (lactase) that is made in your intestinal tract and is required to break down lactose that you ingest. If you are deficient in this enzyme, your intestinal tract struggles to break down and process the milk sugars. This condition is not dangerous, just unpleasant, and most people, even children, will learn to avoid the foods that cause the discomfort—the bloating, the cramping, the reactive diarrhea. For these children, their body is intolerant to milk, but not allergic (allergic would mean that the child's body develops antibodies against milk because it perceives it to be a foreign invader; symptoms include eczema or hives, vomiting, diarrhea, and ear infections).

## A SHORT HISTORY OF MILK

There are two ways that mammals drink milk. One is through breast milk, a natural source of nutrition for all infant mammals. The second option is to drink another mammal's milk. Humans are the only mammals that do this on a regular basis. And they've been doing it for thousands of years, drinking milk mainly from cows, but also from goats, sheep, yaks, water buffalo, and camels. They've also processed this milk into dairy products including cheese, butter, yogurt, kefir (fermented milk), and ice cream. Humans are also the only mammals that continue to consume milk, in whatever form, past their infant years.

People probably began drinking milk when they began domesticating animals. Goats and sheep were domesticated in the area now known as Iran and Afghanistan in about 9000 B.C., and by about 7000 B.C. cattle were being herded in what is now Turkey and parts of Africa. The ancient Greeks and Romans were familiar with methods for making cheese from milk, and from there the use of milk and milk products spread throughout Europe.

What's interesting is that early man (Neolithic period) seems to have been missing the necessary genes to produce the enzyme called lactase, which breaks down lactose, one of the main sugars milk contains. Without this gene, drinking milk can cause bloating, stomach cramps, and diarrhea. As dairy farming evolved, so did the genetic mutation allowing the digestion of milk. And even though nowadays more than 90 percent of people of northern European origin have the necessary gene, intolerance to milk remains a relatively common problem.

## WHAT'S SO GOOD ABOUT MILK?

You may not realize that there is a lot of controversy about milk in this country. Most of us just accept the fact that milk does a body good. And in many ways, it does. A 2009 study from the University of Reading, England found that drinking milk can lessen the chances of dying from illnesses such as coronary heart disease and stroke by up to 15 to 20 percent.

Milk is a kind of all-in-one package for a variety of nutrients growing children need. It has protein, fat, carbohydrates, vitamins, and minerals. Sure, you can get all of these things from other places, but milk has them all conveniently packaged together for you. Here are some of the nutritional benefits of an 8-ounce glass of milk:

- **Calcium:** An 8-ounce serving of milk provides 30 percent of the Daily Value of calcium.

- **Vitamin D:** When fortified, a glass of milk provides about 25 percent of the Daily Value for vitamin D. Vitamin D helps promote the absorption of calcium and enhances bone mineralization.

- **Protein:** An 8-ounce glass of milk provides about 16 percent of the Daily Value for protein. The protein in milk is high quality, which means it contains all of the essential amino acids in the proportions that the body requires for good health.

- **Carbohydrates:** An 8-ounce glass contains 11 grams of carbs in the form of lactose.

- **Fat:** There are about 8 grams of fat in whole milk, while there are negligible amounts of fat in nonfat milk.

- **Potassium:** A glass of milk provides 11 percent of the Daily Value. Potassium regulates the body's fluid balance and helps maintain normal blood pressure. It's also needed for muscle activity.

- **Vitamin A:** A glass of 2 percent, 1 percent, or fat-free milk provides 10 percent of the Daily Value of vitamin A; a glass of whole milk provides 6 percent.

- **Vitamin B12:** Vitamin B12 helps build red blood cells that carry oxygen from the lungs to working muscles. An 8-ounce glass of milk provides about 13 percent of the Daily Value for this vitamin.

- **Riboflavin (vitamin B2):** Milk is an excellent source of riboflavin, providing 24 percent of the Daily Value.

- **Niacin:** A glass of milk provides 10 percent of the Daily Value for niacin.

- **Phosphorus:** Phosphorus helps strengthen bones and generates energy in the body's cells. Milk is an excellent source of phosphorus, providing 20 percent of the Daily Value.

So what's the problem? If milk is so nutrient-dense, meaning that it has a substantial nutritional value for the number of calories, why shouldn't we drink as much as possible? There are actually many reasons not to drink milk, as you will find out in the rest of this chapter. The main problem is that the nutrients in milk don't come into the body independent of all the extra hormones, additives, preservatives, and other natural and man-made "anti-nutrients" that come with it. It's not as if your body can separate out the vitamin D and calcium from the harmful substances that can adversely affect reproductive, immunological, and cognitive functions.

### LET'S START AT THE BEGINNING

Human breast milk is a wondrous thing. Every time a woman breast-feeds her infant, she delivers antibodies that help boost the baby's immune system and keep him safe from all kinds of diseases. The antibodies to specific germs that she has built up over the years are transferred to her baby through each feeding. If you can't breast-feed, the next best option is formula. Companies that make formula have spent millions of dollars creating what is essentially simulated breast milk with all the added nutrients babies need. (Giving your baby cow's milk—at least for the first year of life—is not an option.)

> **The main problem is that the nutrients in milk don't come into the body independent of all the extra hormones, additives, preservatives, and other natural and man-made "anti-nutrients" that come with it.**

Cow's milk is also a wondrous thing—for cows. A 2009 study published in *Genome Biology* looked into the evolution of the milk of various species. University of California Davis researchers reported that they found that "milk proteins that remained the same across species were those proteins related to secreting milk in mammals. Conversely, those milk proteins that had diverged the most from species to species were those associated with the nutritional and immunological components of milk. This suggests that the immunological component of milk is tailored to the particular needs of each species . . ." In other words, the immune-boosting factors in cow's milk are of great help to baby cows but won't do much for baby humans.

**The immune-boosting factors in cow's milk are of great help to baby cows but won't do much for baby humans.**

In fact, the American Academy of Pediatrics advises against using cow's milk as the primary beverage in infants under one year of age. The proteins in cow's milk make it difficult for the baby's immature kidneys to function properly, and the cow's milk proteins are difficult to digest.

If you give milk to children ages one to three years, be sure it's whole milk, not low-fat or nonfat. The greatest time of brain development in a child is from birth until the age of three, and the number one requirement for brain growth is high-quality fat. These days, parents are so worried about their children being overweight that they start to feed them skim milk when they're two or three years old. Don't do it! Check out Chapter 9 for sources of appropriate high-quality fat for toddlers and young children. In the meantime, it is safe to introduce yogurt and cottage cheese (full fat, of course) after the age of one.

---

### Looking for Yogurt? Here Are Some Suggestions

We recommend you look for organic yogurt and cottage cheese for your toddlers: Here are some of our favorite brands:

- Stonyfield Farm Organic Yogurt

- YoBaby Yogurt

- YoKid Yogurt

- Wallaby Organic Yogurt

- Fage Total Yogurt

- Horizon Organic Cottage Cheese

---

After the age of three, kids can drink lower-fat milk if they like. However, we believe that one 8-ounce glass of milk a day is plenty. Remember that your child is probably getting milk from sources other than a straightforward glassful—there's milk in their morning cereal, in the cheese they eat on pizza, in the ice cream they have for dessert. So there's no need to have a glass of milk with every meal.

## THE TROUBLE WITH MILK:
## MILK ALLERGIES AND LACTOSE INTOLERANCE

A small percentage of children—estimates vary from 1 to 7 percent—have an actual allergy to milk. If your child is allergic, it means that her immune system has a negative response to the protein in milk, and she may react with hives, difficulty breathing, or even life-threatening anaphylactic shock. Symptoms are rarely that severe; they mostly range from diarrhea to ear infections to chronic runny nose and cough. The allergic reaction can also cause serious irritation to the intestinal lining, resulting in bleeding, which can in turn cause anemia in infants and toddlers. Milk allergies tend to run in families; if you were allergic to milk as a baby, chances are much higher your baby will be, too. There is no reliable testing for milk allergy, and there is no cure or treatment except to eliminate all milk and dairy products from the diet. The good news is most children outgrow this allergy by the age of two or three.

A much more common condition is known as *lactose intolerance*. Scientists have estimated that about 75 percent of the world's adult population is lactose intolerant. Lactose intolerance is especially prevalent among Asians, Hispanics, Native Americans, and African Americans.

### Oz's Adventures in Dairyland

One thing I remember about my childhood is that I was always sick. I had lots of colds and often suffered from digestive problems. I never thought about why this was happening; it was normal for me. Then, as an adolescent and a young adult, I began to lose my taste for milk and, without thinking about it much, basically eliminated it from my diet. When I was about nineteen, I joined the Youth Corp, a program for urban teens, and worked for them as a summer school teacher. Since school lunches were provided—including milk, of course—I started drinking milk again. Every day. And suddenly I developed horrible stomachaches and gas pains and congestion, and I couldn't understand it. This went on for the better part of the summer. When summer school was over and school lunches were no longer part of my routine, I stopped drinking milk. The digestive problems cleared up immediately. Finally, I put two and two together and realized that maybe milk was the problem. I didn't find out until years later that I was lactose intolerant and probably had been for years.

Being lactose intolerant is very different from being allergic to milk. Whereas a milk allergy involves an immune system response to the whey or casein (proteins) in milk, lactose intolerance does not involve the immune system at all. Lactose is a sugar, made up of glucose and galactose, found in milk. In order to break down this sugar in our bodies, which is necessary so that it can be absorbed through the intestinal wall, we need an enzyme called lactase. We all have this enzyme when we are born, but its production declines, to one degree or another, as we get older. Some people lose the ability to make lactase by the age of three, some in their twenties or thirties, and some never at all.

When people who are lactose intolerant (meaning they are deficient in the lactase enzyme) consume a large amount of food containing lactose, the sugar in it travels undigested through the stomach and into the intestines. It then becomes fermented and can cause symptoms including bloating, gas, cramps, loose stools, and watery diarrhea.

What constitutes a "large amount" can differ from person to person. Your teenager may have no problem eating a cheeseburger even though he gets bloated and gassy if he drinks a glass of milk on its own. For some adults who can't eat a bowl of ice cream without suffering stomach pains, having a small amount of milk in a cup of coffee is not a problem. Drinking milk or eating dairy as part of a meal often makes it easier to digest as well. And many people who can't drink milk can tolerate yogurt and aged cheese because they are somewhat predigested.

In years past, there was only one way to deal with lactose intolerance, and that was to avoid milk and dairy products altogether. These days, lactose-reduced milk is available in many supermarkets and health food stores. You can also take lactase enzyme supplements such as Lactaid and Lacteeze (both are safe for children in recommended doses) to prevent symptoms when consuming lactose-containing dairy products.

---

### Tolerable Snacks

The Dairy Council of California suggests several snacks, eaten in moderation, that can often be enjoyed even by people who are lactose intolerant:

- Whole-grain crackers with Swiss or cheddar cheese slices.

- Plain yogurt combined with dry soup mix as a tasty dip for freshly cut vegetables like carrots, cucumbers, broccoli, and green or red peppers.

- A colorful parfait made of layers of a crumbled bran muffin, sliced fruit, and plain yogurt in a clear bowl, glass, or cup.

---

### *Which Foods Contain the Most Lactose?*

Not all dairy products are created equal. The list below is a sampling of some of the highest lactose-containing food sources:

| | | |
|---|---|---|
| Fat-free dry milk | ⅓ cup | 12 g |
| Milk: whole, low-fat, skim | 1 cup | 9 to 12 g |
| Buttermilk | 1 cup | 9 to 12 g |
| Ice cream | ½ cup | 6 g |

| | | |
|---|---|---|
| Yogurt, low-fat | 1 cup | 5 g |
| Condensed milk, whole | 2 tbsp. | 4 g |
| Sour cream | ½ cup | 4 g |
| Evaporated milk | 1 tbsp. | 3 g |
| Cottage cheese | ½ cup | 2 to 3 g |
| Sherbet | ½ cup | 2 g |
| Cheese: American, Swiss, blue | 1 oz. | 1 to 2 g |
| Cheese: cheddar, Parmesan | 1 oz. | 1 to 2 g |
| Cream cheese | 1 oz. | 1 to 2 g |
| Whipped cream | 2 tbsp. | <1 g |
| Butter or margarine | 1 cup | trace |

According to the Center for Food Allergies in Seattle (www .centerforfoodallergies.com), there are many hidden sources of lactose you should be aware of if you're lactose intolerant, including:

- Artificial sweeteners containing lactose

- Breads, biscuits, and crackers, doughnuts made with milk

- Breading on fried foods

- Breakfast and baby cereals containing milk solids

- Buttered or creamed foods (soups and vegetables)

- Cake and pudding mixes, many frostings

- Candies with milk chocolate

- Cookies made with milk

- Hot dogs, luncheon meats, sausage, hash, processed and canned meats

- Mayonnaise and salad dressings made with milk

- Nondairy creamers (except for Coffee Rich)

- Pancakes, waffles, toaster tarts

- Pizza

- Foods containing whey, casein, caseinate, or sodium caseinate

## MORE TROUBLE WITH MILK: MEDICAL PROBLEMS DOWN THE LINE

In previous chapters on carbs, corn, and wheat, we stated that much of the problems with these foods arise from the fact that they just aren't what they used to be—for the most part, they're no longer natural foods eaten in their purest forms. The same can be said for milk. We're not talking about milk that's come directly from the cow to you. And we're not talking about the cow that grazed in the back 40, either. We're talking about a highly manipulated food product called milk that comes from animals that have been fed hormones, antibiotics, and numerous other chemicals that enter our nutrient stream every time we swallow it down.

And, as with carbs, corn, and wheat, the problem isn't so much that we drink milk and eat dairy products, it's that we guzzle and devour so much of these products. To the extent that milk should ever be consumed at all, it was never meant to be consumed in the amounts we consume it now.

Studies have shown that the overconsumption and manipulation of milk and milk products are causing children to have a variety of health problems as they get older. Many of these studies are controversial and most scientists agree that more research needs to be conducted before definitive results can be claimed. However, it's worth noting what some of those problems are:

- **Diabetes:** Juvenile-onset or type 1 diabetes is caused when the body's immune system attacks and destroys insulin-producing cells in the pancreas. Cow's milk may have something to do with this. Researchers found that diabetics have a much higher than normal level of antibodies to a protein in cow's milk called bovine serum albumin, which turns out to be remarkably similar to a protein on the surface of insulin-producing cells. The antibodies that have been formed to fight the cow's protein then mistakenly attack and destroy the lookalike insulin-producing cells.

- **Asthma:** It has long been assumed that milk exacerbated asthma by stimulating mucus production in the lungs. However, new research is finding that undiagnosed milk allergies may be the underlying problem behind the link between milk and asthma. Milk allergies often disappear as children get older; this may explain why asthma sometimes disappears as well.

- **Human reproductive disorders:** Many studies have found that the hormones found in milk and milk products are affecting human reproduction in a variety of ways. The reason, researchers say, is that because of advanced milking technologies, dairy farmers now milk their cows about 300 days per year. The cows are pregnant for much of that time, and as the pregnancy progresses, production of estrogen increases. That estrogen is then passed along into the milk we drink.

In addition to their natural hormones, dairy cows are often injected with recombinant Bovine Growth Hormone (rBGH) in order to increase milk production. This has caused a number of problems. First, rBGH is known to cause inflammation in cows' udders. Traces of the antibiotics used to treat this problem then get into our milk supply.

Some scientists have posited that for prepubescent boys, high milk and dairy consumption might interfere with physiological development of the reproductive system and result in decreased semen quality in adulthood. Cow's milk has also been associated with early sexual maturity. It has long been noted that young people, especially girls, are reaching sexual maturity younger and younger. After World War II, dairy products, which had never been a significant part of the Japanese diet, were introduced into the country's diet by occupying American troops. According to studies, the per capita yearly dietary intake of dairy products in 1950 was only 5.5 pounds. Twenty-five years later, the average Japanese consumed 117.4 pounds of milk and dairy products. In 1950, the average twelve-year-old Japanese girl was 4 feet 6 inches tall, weighed 71 pounds, and had her first period at the age of fifteen. By 1975, the average Japanese girl, who by now was consuming a variety of milk and dairy products, was 5 feet 5 inches tall, weighed 90 pounds, and had her first period at the age of twelve.

Milk has also been linked to acne, autism, ADHD, and many other diseases and conditions, including cancer. In some cases, these claims have been made on the basis of one or two studies, and the risks involved have been deemed small. Right now, no one knows for sure the harm milk does. So what are you to do? Remember our credo: Moderation is the key. A glass of milk, some cheese and crackers, or a few scoops of ice cream now and then will not significantly affect your child's health. Having them all together or all in one day might not be the best choice; a better idea may be to manage your child's diet so that a dairy overload does not become a problem.

---

### Go Organic

If you're going to serve cow's milk, try certified organic milk. It doesn't contain antibiotics or bovine growth hormone. Buying organic can be costly. If you are on a budget and you have to choose which organic products to buy, here's our advice: Buy organic dairy, beef, and chicken, especially if you have prepubescent children. Be sure to look for "organic," not just "antibiotic-free." If it says "organic" it means it doesn't have growth hormones or other additives. Then buy the freshest produce you can afford, even if it's not organic (frozen fruits and vegetables are healthy for you as well). Just be sure to wash the produce well.

---

## IF NOT MILK, THEN WHAT?

Many parents are afraid to stop giving their children dairy products because they don't know how else to make sure they're getting enough calcium. According to the International Food Information Council, more than half of American children and teens do not meet their daily calcium requirements. The National Institutes of Health (NIH) lists the recommended daily allowance (RDA) of calcium as follows:

| Birth to 6 months | 210 mg |
|---|---|
| 7 to 12 months | 270 mg |
| 1 to 3 years | 500 mg |
| 4 to 8 years | 800 mg |
| 9 to 13 years | 1300 mg |
| 14 to 18 years | 1300 mg |
| 19 to 50 years | 1000 mg |

The good news is that many other foods besides dairy products contain calcium. Some of them are foods kids love to eat; others, not so much. On the other hand, you may be surprised what your kids will eat if you don't make a big deal out of it, and if you eat it as well. Sardines, anyone? The list below includes some of the best sources of calcium:

| Plain low-fat yogurt | 8 oz. | 415 mg |
|---|---|---|
| Sardines, canned in oil with bones | 3 oz. | 324 mg |
| Cheddar cheese | 1.5 oz. | 306 mg |
| Sesame seeds | 1 oz. | 280 mg |
| Orange juice, calcium-fortified | 6 oz. | 200 to 260 mg |
| Pink salmon, canned | 3 oz. | 181 mg |
| Cottage cheese, 1 percent | 1 cup | 138 mg |
| Spinach, cooked | ½ cup | 120 mg |
| Frozen yogurt, vanilla soft serve | ½ cup | 103 mg |
| Cereal, calcium-fortified | ½ cup | 100 to 200 mg |
| Kale, cooked | 1 cup | 94 mg |
| Almonds | 1 oz. | 80 mg |
| Broccoli, chopped | ½ cup | 47 mg |

### Drinkable Alternatives

For many of us, there was nothing as comforting as coming home from school to a snack of a couple of cookies and an ice-cold glass of milk. Kids still crave the same thing, so what can you give them to drink if you don't want to go with the milk of the cow?

- **Try the milk of the goat.** In many areas of the world, goat's milk is the drink of choice. Although we protested earlier about not drinking another mammal's milk, many children find goat's milk is more easily digestible and less allergenic than cow's milk. Goat's milk also contains slightly less lactose (4.1 percent versus 4.7 percent in cow's milk). However, goat's milk contains less folic acid (which is important in the production of normal red blood cells and for preventing heart disease, stroke, and certain cancers) than cow's milk, so be sure to buy goat's milk that says "fortified with folic acid" on the label.

- **Try rice milk:** It is certainly okay to give your kids rice milk to drink, but it's important to note that it does not have the same kind of nutrient values of either cow's or goat's milk. In fact, it can't legally be called milk as that term is reserved exclusively for dairy products. Since it's made from rice, it's a source of carbohydrates rather than the proteins, fats, and carbs of cow's and goat's milk. Rice milk is not a good substitute if you're not making any other adjustments in your children's diet. However, you might want to try a product like Rice Dream, a nondairy ice cream–like frozen dessert.

### What About Soy Milk?

Many parents who are concerned about the harmful effects of cow's milk turn to soy milk as a healthy alternative. But soy may not be as healthy as we have been led to believe. The main concern about soy formula is that it contains high levels of phytoestrogens—estrogen-like substances found in some plants. For that reason, we do not recommend soy milk as a substitute for cow's milk.

# Questions to Ask Your Child's Doctor

- Can you tell if my daughter is lactose intolerant? Could she have a milk allergy?

- Is my baby growing well enough to restrict his milk intake? What alternatives to milk can you recommend?

- How old should my baby be before I introduce yogurt to her diet?

- I know I should not give my child cow's milk before he turns one, but what about cheese and other forms of dairy?

- My baby is in the 95th percentile for weight and only the 50th for height. When is it okay to give her skim milk?

- My family has a history of milk allergy. What should I start my baby on once I stop breast-feeding?

- I am allergic to milk. Can you advise me on a nonmilk alternative, since I want to have good nutrition for my breast milk?

- Will dry or powdered milk also cause allergy?

- My nine-month-old is allergic to milk. I have not been giving him milk or dairy products. His symptoms are much improved, but they still come back every once in a while. Why is that?

- Is LACTAID milk safe to give my child even if I am not sure he is lactose intolerant?

# Chapter 7 Take-Home Points

- Lactose intolerance and milk allergy are not the same. Lactose intolerance is a deficiency in the lactase enzyme needed to break down lactose that you ingest. A milk allergy involves an immune system response to the whey or casein (proteins) in milk.

- Humans are also the only mammals that continue to consume milk, in whatever form, past their infant years.

- Early man (Neolithic period) seems to have been missing the necessary genes to produce the lactase enzyme. It was only with the evolution of dairy farming that a genetic mutation occurred in humans, allowing the digestion of milk. Though nowadays more than 90 percent of people of northern European origin have the necessary gene, intolerance to milk remains a relatively common problem.

- The American Academy of Pediatrics advises against using cow's milk as the primary beverage in infants under one year of age. The proteins in cow's milk make it difficult for the baby's immature kidneys to function properly, and the cow's milk proteins are difficult to digest.

- If you give milk to children ages one to three years, be sure it's whole milk, not low-fat or nonfat.

- One 8-ounce glass of milk a day is plenty. Your child is probably getting milk from other sources as well, so there's no need to have a glass of milk with every meal.

- A small percentage of children have an actual allergy to milk. This means that a child's immune system has a negative response to the protein in milk, and she may react with hives, difficulty breathing, or even life-threatening anaphylactic shock.

- Milk allergies tend to run in families; if you were allergic to milk as a baby, chances are much higher your baby will be, too. Most children outgrow this allergy by the age of two or three.

- The milk we get from stores today is a highly manipulated food product that comes from animals that have been fed hormones, antibiotics, and numerous other chemicals that enter our nutrient stream every time we drink it.

- Studies have shown that the overconsumption and manipulation of milk and milk products are causing children to have a variety of health problems as they get older, including diabetes, asthma, reproductive disorders, and cancer.

- Goat's milk, fortified with folic acid, may be a viable substitute for cow's milk.

As we've said all along, there's no need to totally eliminate dairy products unless your child is truly allergic. But if you did eliminate this food group from your child's diet, he or she could still survive and thrive (perhaps with the help of some specific supplements, as you'll see in Chapter 11). The same cannot be said for the next food group: proteins. Proteins are our bodies' fundamental building blocks. They are found in every cell in our bodies. Luckily for us, proteins are found in many different kinds of foods, so whether your child is a meat eater or a vegetarian, there will always be something to eat and enjoy.

# CHAPTER 8

# Let's Get Specific: Protein

*What are little boys made of?*
*Snips and snails*
*and puppy dog tails.*
*That's what little boys are made of.*

*What are little girls made of?*
*Sugar and spice*
*and everything nice.*
*That's what little girls are made of.*

Take a look at your child. What do you see? Underneath the sugar and spice, snips and snails and puppy dog tails, cute-as-can-be exterior is an essential structure that enables your child to stand, walk, grow, breathe, circulate blood, and digest food. That structure is made of protein, one of three major classes of nutrients that provide calories to the body (the other two are carbohydrates and fats). Proteins are part of every cell in your body—they're in your muscles, your bones, your blood, your organs, your skin, and your hair; they're in your antibodies, enzymes, and hormones. They are used to build, repair, and replace every tissue in your body.

Proteins differ from carbohydrates and fats in one very important way: You don't have to spend time worrying about proteins that are bad for you. There are no unhealthy proteins. When we warn against eating too much red meat, for instance, it's not the protein portion we're concerned about. It's the carbohydrates (remember that most of the beef produced today is full of corn) and the fat (saturated), which is why we recommend choosing lean organic meat. You can't really eat too

**There are no unhealthy proteins.**

much protein. If you eat more than is necessary (we'll get to adequate amounts later), the excess is eliminated through the kidneys. The body doesn't store protein the way it stores fat.

## WHY DO YOUR KIDS NEED PROTEIN?

Proteins are fundamental components of all living cells. That pretty much says it all. Every part and system of our body needs protein to function. Besides building, repairing, and replacing tissue, protein helps to stabilize blood sugar, enabling us to burn more sugar between meals. It also keeps us full longer (and more likely to stay away from the munchies).

Children who don't get enough protein do not grow and develop as they should. Protein helps the body to produce a number of important chemicals used to create antibodies, enzymes, and hormones. Your body needs protein to regenerate hair and nails. All of the body's responses require that your body makes protein, whether it's protein to rebuild tissue, to heal wounds, or to fight infection.

## AMINO ACIDS: THE BUILDING BLOCKS OF PROTEINS

If our cells are made mostly of proteins, what are proteins made of? The answer is amino acids, small molecules that link together in long chains to form proteins. The proteins you eat are broken down by the digestive system into amino acids. Those amino acids are then recombined to make thousands of different proteins, which are subsequently used by the body to maintain and repair tissues, blood, and bone. Have your kids ever played with Lego blocks? Imagine that your child builds a fortress of Legos, then knocks it over and reassembles those same blocks into a pirate ship. The same thing happens with amino acids in the body. Proteins come into your body, are "disassembled" into individual amino acids, and then reassembled into proteins again.

There are actually several hundred amino acids, but only about twenty-two of them are important to human health. Out of those twenty-two, nine are known as essential amino acids. That means, like essential fatty acids, your body can't make them, so you have to get them from the foods you eat. No matter how healthy you are, you cannot produce these nine amino acids, so it is literally essential that you get them from an external source.

Proteins are organized into different categories according to how many of the essential amino acids they provide:

> No matter how healthy you are, you cannot produce these nine amino acids, so it is literally essential that you get them from an external source.

- **Complete proteins:** A complete protein contains all nine essential amino acids. Since animal tissues contain amino acids similar to our own, foods that come from animals (e.g., meat, eggs, cheese) contain complete proteins.

- **Incomplete proteins:** These proteins, which include most vegetable proteins, are missing one or more essential amino acids.

- **Complementary proteins:** When you combine two or more incomplete sources of protein, they will provide adequate amounts of the essential amino acids you need. For instance, you can serve peanut butter (made from peanuts, an incomplete vegetable protein) with whole grain bread, another incomplete source of protein, and you've got a complete protein. Or cook some red or black beans, mix them with brown rice, and voilà! Another complete protein.

---

### Variety Is the Source of Life

Not too long ago, when nutritionists advised that complementary proteins needed to be eaten together, they meant together at the same meal. Current wisdom, however, has revised that theory. The good news is that you don't have to provide your child with all nine essential amino acids at every meal. As long as he eats a variety of proteins throughout the day, the amino acids will combine

---

to give him what he needs. So if you want to serve him oatmeal at breakfast and black-eyed peas with dinner, feel free. You've got your family covered as far as proteins are concerned.

Here are some sample combinations that form a complete protein:

- Legumes (edible seeds or pods such as beans, lentils, and peas) with grains

- Legumes with nuts

- Legumes with seeds

- Grains with dairy

- Nuts/seeds with dairy

- Legumes with dairy

## CHOOSING HEALTHY PROTEINS

Parents are often worried because they think their children are not getting enough protein. That's because they usually equate protein with chicken and beef. But many foods besides poultry and red meat are high in protein, which means that your kids are likely getting much more protein in their diet than you think. Proteins are in abundance around us. They are found in the following foods:

- Meat (beef, pork, venison, and other game animals)

- Poultry

- Fish

- Legumes

- Eggs

- Nuts and seeds

- Milk, yogurt, and cheese

- Grains

We advocate for more animal protein for children, such as from fish, yogurt, eggs, lean cuts of meat, organic chicken, and organic turkey. Making things a little more complicated, protein requirements also depend on the quality of protein your child eats and how easily digestible it is.

The best foods to eat for protein are not necessarily those that are highest in grams of protein, but those that are highest in quality. In general, animal proteins are considered highly digestible and higher quality than plant sources of protein, in part because plant sources also have a lot more fiber, which is indigestible. It's not that plant protein is not as good, per se, it's just that you'd have to eat so much of it. You'd have to consume humongous amounts of kale or broccoli, for instance, to get the same amount of protein as you'd find in a small serving of steak. You don't have to worry about this though, as long as you vary the protein foods your child eats.

Here are some tips about choosing quality proteins:

> **The best foods to eat for protein are not necessarily those that are highest in grams of protein, but those that are highest in quality. In general, animal proteins are considered highly digestible and higher quality than plant sources of protein, in part because plant sources also have a lot more fiber, which is indigestible.**

**Choose the leanest cuts of meat you can find.**
- Look for the words "loin" or "round" in the name. The seven leanest cuts are eye round, top round, round tip, top sirloin, bottom round, top loin, and tenderloin. If you're buying ground beef, look for ground sirloin or ground round, and choose packages labeled lean or extra lean. Of course, these cuts

of meat, especially if you're buying organic, are the most expensive. So buy the best cut of meat you can afford.

- Packaged meat will also contain a grade on the label. The most common grades are prime, choice, and select. The highest grade is prime, which means that the meat has the most marbling, or streaks of fat, and is therefore very tender. Select has the least amount of marbling and is consequently less tender. A good way to tenderize a lean cut of meat is to marinate it for at least six hours in a blend of an acidic ingredient such as vinegar, wine, or citrus juice with a little bit of olive oil, herbs, and spices.

**Chicken and turkey are always good choices.**

- Cutting off the excess fat and removing the skin are the healthiest ways to go. But don't forget that there are many ways to serve poultry. You can get lean ground chicken and ground turkey for healthy alternative-style burgers, meat loaf, or meat sauce. Chicken and turkey can also be used in chili, tacos, and most other dishes that are traditionally made with ground beef.

**Fish is a naturally lean source of protein.**

- Seafood is especially good because of the relationship between omega-3 fatty acids that are found in fish and seafood and the development of children's brains and immune systems. However, children don't usually gobble down a salmon fillet at first taste; they often have to be coaxed into eating fish at all. The easiest way to help them learn to enjoy fish is for them to watch you enjoying it, too. It's best to start your kids on a mild tasting fish first. Although fish like salmon have the highest omega-3 fatty acids, they also have the strongest flavor. Start eating white fish like grouper or Vietnamese basa fillets and gradually work your way up to salmon.

- There are some caveats about feeding fish to children, however. The American College of Allergy, Asthma, and Immunology puts fish on its list of most common food allergens, and recommends that you introduce fish only after your child's first birthday, when his immune and digestive systems are more developed. And there's always the question of mercury overload (see Chapter 9), which is why the U.S. Food and Drug Administration (FDA) recommends that you avoid feeding your child large predatory fish, including shark, swordfish, king mackerel, and tilefish, which contain the highest levels of mercury. You should also stick to light tuna, and limit your child's intake to about 1 ounce of tuna per week for kids weighing up to 20 pounds, and about 3 ounces (half a can of tuna) for kids weighing between 20 and 60 pounds. The American Academy of Pediatrics also warns that children shouldn't eat raw or undercooked fish, which may contain bacteria and viruses that can be tolerated by healthy adults but can make young children seriously ill.

**Eggs are an almost perfect food.**

- They are rich in nutrients, both in amino acids as well as key vitamins and minerals. Egg whites are almost pure protein. Your kids can eat as many egg whites per week as they like, but because egg yolks contain cholesterol, the standard recommendation is to limit whole eggs to three per week.

- Eggs are one of those foods where buying organic does make a difference. Tests have shown that organic eggs have, on average, one-third less cholesterol than commercial eggs. They also have four to six times the vitamin D, one-quarter less saturated fat, two times more omega-3 fatty acid, and three times more vitamin E.

- Remember that eggs should always be cooked thoroughly. Raw eggs are breeding places for salmonella. Federal researchers estimate that more than 130,000 people are sickened every year and 30 die as a result of contaminated eggs.

## How Much Protein Do Kids Need?

Even if your child is in a stage where he won't eat meat or fish, there is really no need to worry about whether or not he or she is getting enough protein. According to the American Academy of Pediatrics, "protein is so abundant in the foods Americans eat, that most of us, children and adults alike, consume more than we need." This is especially true since only 10 to 30 percent of our daily calories should come from protein. The amount of protein necessary for the body's growth and maintenance depends on your child's age. The Recommended Dietary Allowances (RDA) for different age groups are as follows:

| Age | Grams of Protein Needed Each Day* |
|-----|-----------------------------------|
| 1 to 3 | 13 |
| 4 to 8 | 19 |
| 9 to 13 | 34 |
| 14 to 18 (girls) | 46 |
| 14 to 18 (boys) | 52 |

*There are 7 grams in 1 ounce of protein.

### How Much Protein Is in My Food?

If you're looking at a canned or packaged food, the number of protein grams per serving will be on the label. If you want to know how many grams are in unpackaged foods, you can go to the Web site for the National Agricultural Library (www.nal.usda.gov). You'll find a huge list of foods and their protein grams. Here is just a sampling:

| | | |
|---|---|---|
| Chicken | 1 cup | 43 g |
| Halibut | ½ fillet | 43 g |
| Salmon | 5 oz. | 42 g |
| Turkey | 1 cup | 41 g |

| | | |
|---|---|---|
| Pork loin | 3 oz. | 27 g |
| Roast beef | 3 oz. | 26 g |
| Cottage cheese, nonfat | 1 cup | 25 g |
| Tuna, light, in oil, drained | 3 oz. | 25 g |
| Ground beef | 3 oz. | 22 g |
| Couscous | 1 cup | 22 g |
| Tuna, white, in water | 3 oz. | 20 g |
| Lentils | 1 cup | 18 g |
| Lima beans | 1 cup | 15 g |
| Chickpeas | 1 cup | 15 g |
| Yogurt, low-fat | 1 cup | 12 g |
| Peas | 8 oz. | 8 g |
| Peanuts, dry roasted | 1 oz. | 7 g |
| Egg | 1 large | 6 g |
| Spinach, cooked | 1 cup | 5g |
| Rice, brown, cooked | 1 cup | 5g |
| Peanut butter | 1 tbsp. | 4g |

## GET TO KNOW YOUR BS AND QS

If you're looking to add variety to your menu of proteins, don't forget your Bs and Qs: beans and quinoa. Many beans are a wonderful source of protein and are especially critical for those choosing a vegetarian diet (plus they're loaded with valuable fiber). Lentils are a particularly good choice because 1 cup has 17 grams of protein with only .75 grams of fat. A 2-ounce extra-lean sirloin steak has the same amount of protein but six times the fat. Some other healthy beans include black beans, chickpeas, kidney beans, garbanzo beans, and legumes, to name a few. It's best to soak dried beans overnight before preparing them in any dish because beans can cause your kids to have digestive problems. For children twelve years and older, you can also try products like Beano, a natural food enzyme dietary supplement that can help prevent gas before it starts.

Quinoa, a South American grain, is one of the few complete plant proteins. Although it is usually categorized as a grain, technically it is a seed that is rich in essential fats, vitamins, and minerals and an excellent source of calcium, iron, and vitamins B and E.

You cook quinoa much as you cook rice: Bring 2 cups of water to a boil with 1 cup of quinoa; cover at a low simmer and cook for 14 to 18 minutes or until the germ separates from the seed. The cooked germ looks like a tiny curl and should have a slight bite to it (like al dente pasta). Quinoa has a slightly nutty flavor and can be a great breakfast treat for you and your kids, especially when you add some fresh berries and a small amount of rice or almond milk, and sweeten with honey. Delicious.

The whole idea is to eat as much of a variety of proteins as possible. If you eat only one protein source, you limit the number of amino acids you will consume. If you were to feed your child three meals a day made up entirely of convenient processed fast foods, he might get the full range of calories he should have for the day, but you would not be providing him with the essential proteins and other nutrients he requires for healthy growth and development. If you want to get the most effective performance out of your child, he or she needs to be exposed to a complete pool of amino acids on a regular basis. Every organ and organ system, every hormone, every brain, muscle, and bone cell pivots on the introduction and rotation of all the different amino acids that are found in proteins.

# Questions to Ask Your Child's Doctor

- Does the amount of protein my child needs vary with age or activity level?

- My child lives on pizza and chicken nuggets. Does that count as enough protein?

- Are there any proteins I should not give my children because of the cholesterol history in my family?

- We are vegetarians, so my child gets his protein only from plant sources, not animals. How can I be sure he's getting enough protein?

# Chapter 8 Take-Home Points

- Proteins are part of every cell in your body—they're in your muscles, your bones, your blood, your organs, your skin, and your hair; they're in your antibodies, enzymes, and hormones. They are used to build, repair, and replace every tissue in your body.

- Unlike fats and carbohydrates, there are no unhealthy proteins.

- Children who don't get enough protein do not grow and develop as they should. If they are deprived of protein for any length of time, their immune system will weaken and they will be unable to fight off disease and infection.

- Proteins are made up of amino acids, small molecules that link together in long chains to form proteins. The proteins you eat are broken down by the digestive system into amino acids. Those amino acids are then recombined to make thousands of different proteins, which are subsequently used by the body to maintain and repair tissues, blood, and bone.

- Proteins are organized into different categories according to how many of the essential amino acids they provide: complete proteins, which contain all nine essential amino acids (these come from animal sources); incomplete proteins, which include most vegetable proteins and are missing one or more essential amino acids; and complementary proteins, which are formed when you combine two or more incomplete sources of protein.

- In general, animal proteins are considered highly digestible and higher quality than plant sources of protein. You don't have to worry about this though, as long as you vary the protein foods your child eats.

- Make sure your children eat a wide variety of proteins so that they will get the whole complement of amino acids. There is no need to worry about whether your child is getting enough protein since most Americans consume more protein than we need. This is especially true since only 10 to 30 percent of our daily calories should come from protein.

While the fact that most Americans get more protein than we need is not particularly harmful to our well-being, the fact that most Americans get more fat than we need may be detrimental to our health. But what most of us don't know is that not all fat is bad for us—in fact, for children fat is absolutely essential to proper growth and development. The trick is to know which fats are good for their health, and which fats are not. The next chapter will tell you everything you need to know.

# Chapter 9

# Let's Get Specific: Fats

Nothing seems to concern and confuse people more, nutritionally speaking, than the "F" word. The word "fat" strikes fear into the hearts of anyone concerned about health—their own or their loved ones'. Parents are afraid that feeding their children fat will make their children overweight. And in some respects, they're right.

It takes energy to digest, absorb, and assimilate the various nutrients from any food we take in. This process burns more calories from protein and carbohydrate than it does with fat. About 23 out of every 100 calories from protein, for example, are burned in the process of absorbing nutrients. Fat, on the other hand, comes into the body almost in the form in which it can be stored. We use only about 3 out of every 100 calories of fat to adapt it to the form in which it resides on our thighs. If one day you ate 2,000 calories of fat, it probably made you heavier than if you ate 2,000 calories of carbohydrate or protein.

**More than a third of a child's caloric intake should be made up of fat. But not just any fat.**

But children need fat for their growth and development. In fact, more than a third of a child's caloric intake should be made up of fat. But not just any fat. It's important that the fat, as much as possible, should come from healthy sources such as avocados and omega-3 fish oils. This chapter will introduce these healthy fats, explain the difference between essential fatty acids, saturated fats, unsaturated fats, and trans fatty acid, and lay out the best and worst fats to feed your kids. We're going to help you navigate through the pros and cons of fats in your children's diets.

## HEALTHY VS. UNHEALTHY FATS

The first thing to know is that certain classes of fat are very important to human health. There's a definite link between these fats and healthy development of the brain and the body, including cognitive, behavioral, and immune system functions. As we get older, the health of the heart and the cardiovascular system is based on the kinds of fats we have had in our diet starting in early childhood. The earlier these good fats are consumed, the better your children will be able to control inflammation, heart disease, mood disorders, and many other health issues as they get older.

On the other hand, there are unhealthy fats, such as partially hydrogenated or trans fatty acids, which we will describe in this chapter, that can be extremely harmful to your child's health if they are overconsumed. And, since these fats are ubiquitous in this country, many children are consuming them in large amounts on a daily basis. Over time, these fats can alter a child's metabolism, as well as their ability to regulate weight and appetite.

What's important for you to understand is that fat is not the enemy. What seems like such a logical concept—eat less fat and you become less fat—is a theory that doesn't hold up. Just look around and you can prove it to yourself. For many years, the American public and—much more damaging—the American food producers have latched onto the "low-fat, no-fat" approach to food consumption as the ultimate answer to weight loss and a healthy heart. If that were true, we'd all be thin and disease-free. But Americans, and especially American kids, are fatter than ever, and heart disease is still the number one cause of death in the United States. So cutting out all the fat can't be the answer.

Fortunately, the past few years have brought about a new understanding of the role of fats in our diet, especially where our children are concerned. What we have discovered is that children need dietary fats for proper growth and development. And we also now know that it's not fat in general that's causing us problems, it's that most of us are ingesting too much of the wrong kinds of fat and too little of the right kinds. The best thing we can do for ourselves and our kids is to learn to tell the difference.

## THE SKINNY ON FATS

All bodily cells need fat to function; it provides fuel for cells. It also helps build cell membranes and the outer layer that surrounds the cell and controls what goes in and out of the cells themselves. It helps create myelin, the protective sheath that covers neurons (nerve cells that send and receive electrical signals within the body); myelin is composed of 30 percent protein and 70 percent fat. And, last but by no means least, about two-thirds of your brain is composed of fats. But not every kind of fat is good for your health. The challenge of any discussion on fat, and one of the reasons the subject is so confusing, is that there are so many different kinds. The definitions below will help you understand the concepts we'll be introducing as this chapter goes on:

- **Essential Fatty Acid (EFA):** A building block of the body necessary for human health. The body cannot make EFAs, so we must get them from the foods we eat (e.g., salmon, sardines, avocados—see page 129 for a list of other EFA-containing foods). There are two kinds of essential fatty acids. The first is alpha-linolenic acid (ALA), which is the foundation of omega-3 fatty acids; the second is linoleic acid (LA), the foundation of omega-6 fatty acids. EFAs are critical for proper growth in children, especially for neural development and maturation of sensory systems. It's also vital that expectant mothers get adequate supplies of EFAs, as they are passed on to fetuses and nursing babies.

- **Omega-3 Fatty Acid:** Omega-3 is a polyunsaturated EFA found in a variety of foods, including fatty fish, flaxseed oil or ground flaxseed, canola oil, walnut oil, and omega-3 fortified eggs (see Chapter 11 on supplements).

- **EPA:** An omega-3 fatty acid known as eicosapentaenoic acid, important in assisting the function of the brain and immune system.

- **DHA:** An omega-3 fatty acid incorporated into neural and eye tissue, docosahexaenoic acid (DHA) is critical for the development and function of the brain, nerve cells, and the eyes. DHA is also important in the function and maintenance of the immune system, hormone regulation, and general health.

- **Omega-6 Fatty Acid:** A polyunsaturated EFA found in green leafy vegetables and in flaxseed, safflower, borage, and evening primrose oils, omega-6 stimulates fat-burning tissue in the body, encouraging calories to be burned for energy instead of being stored as fat.

- **Saturated Fat:** Saturated fat has a large amount of hydrogen attached to it (which is why it is "saturated") and is therefore usually solid at room temperature; it is found in animal fats and in some tropical oils such as coconut and palm.

- **Unsaturated Fat:** This type of fat has fewer hydrogen atoms attached to it (which is why it is *un*saturated). It is derived from plant and some animal sources, especially fish, and is liquid at room temperature. There are two types of this fat: monounsaturated and polyunsaturated.

- **Hydrogenated:** This means that hydrogen has been artificially added to oils at extremely high temperatures to solidify them and give them longer shelf lives. Margarine is probably the most well-known hydrogenated product.

- **Trans Fatty Acid:** The process of hydrogenating fat causes it to change its molecular structure into what is called a trans fatty acid. Although many restaurants, fast food places, and food manufacturers are reducing or eliminating trans fatty acids, they can still be found in many commercially packaged goods, commercially fried food such as french fries from some fast food chains, other packaged snacks such as microwave popcorn, and in vegetable shortening and some margarine. Indeed, any packaged goods that contain "partially hydrogenated vegetable oils," "hydrogenated vegetable oils," or "shortening" most likely contain trans fat. Trans fatty acids increase a product's shelf life, but may decrease yours.

**How Fats Turned Us into Intelligent Human Beings**

According to some theories, fats may have turned us into what we are today. Millions of years ago, animal life originated in the sea, where there is an abundance of omega-3 fatty acids. Time passed, and flowering seed plants containing omega-6 fatty acids appeared on earth. The first humans had brains that were not very developed. Then, about 200,000 years ago, things began to change. Scientists believe that early human populations who lived near water and ate plants and seafood (such as people in the East African Rift Valley and on the southern Cape of South Africa) began to demonstrate a greater intelligence. The theory is that this was due to their diets, which included both omega-3 and omega-6 fatty acids. This plant and seafood diet was particularly rich in DHA, an essential factor in brain development. On the other hand, the brains of the Australopithecines, who lived inland and did not have access to seafood, never developed more than ape-like characteristics.

## WHY THE GOOD FATS ARE GOOD FOR YOU

"Good" fats are those that are least saturated: omega-3s, omega-6s, monounsaturated, and polyunsaturated. The worst fats are the most saturated: hydrogenated, partially hydrogenated, and trans fats.

There are many reasons why good fats are beneficial to your overall health, some of which we mentioned earlier: Fats help fuel the body; fats build healthy cells and cell membranes; fats help create myelin, the insulation that surrounds nerve fibers and makes it easier for nerves to communicate more quickly with each other; and fats build better brains. In addition:

- **Fats protect and cushion your organs.** Many of your most vital organs, including the heart, kidneys, and intestines, are held in place and protected from injury by layers of fat.

- **Fat helps the body absorb vitamins.** Some vitamins—A, D, E, and K—are fat soluble, which means that the fats in foods help the intestines absorb them into the body.

- **Fats are necessary for the manufacturing of hormones,** especially prostaglandins, which help regulate digestion, immune functions, and reproductive activity.

- **Fats help regulate body temperature.**

- **Fat provides a sense of satiety.** Fat helps you feel full longer. For example, if you feed your child an omelet of reduced-fat cheese and egg whites at 7:00 a.m., he may be hungry again before the first school period of the day. But if you take out the reduced-fat cheese and instead use a small portion of Swiss or cheddar, your child may be good to go until lunchtime. That's because fat actually takes longer to digest than other types of foods. Since it sticks around in your stomach a while, your child will feel fuller longer.

- **Fat makes food taste good.** If it wasn't for fats, the food you eat wouldn't taste anywhere near as good as it does. That's why many "fat-free" foods are more fattening than you would think—because they use added sugar to make up for the flavor deficit.

## FAT SUPERSTARS: OMEGA-3, DHA, AND OMEGA-6

Foods that contain these superstar fats should be part of your child's diet as much as possible. Check out the lists of foods below and introduce them slowly into your child's repertoire of foods—the more variety the better.

### Omega-3

Omega-3 fatty acids may play a role in the prevention and/or treatment of the following health conditions:

- Alzheimer's disease

- Asthma

- Attention deficit hyperactivity disorder (ADHD)

- Bipolar disorder

- Cancer

- Cardiovascular disease

- Depression

- Diabetes

- Eczema

- High blood pressure

- Lupus

- Migraine headaches

- Multiple sclerosis

- Obesity

- Osteoarthritis

- Osteoporosis

- Psoriasis

- Rheumatoid arthritis

With a list like that you can see why omega-3s are so important to our health. Some of these conditions may not be of immediate concern to your children (e.g., osteoporosis and Alzheimer's disease), but building up good health habits while they're young may stave off these diseases as they get older.

Some of the best food sources of omega-3s are fatty fish, including:

| | |
|---|---|
| Atlantic mackerel | Salmon |
| Trout | Tuna |
| Herring | Striped bass |
| Sardines | Anchovies |

Other excellent food sources of omega-3s include:

| | |
|---|---|
| Flaxseeds | Avocados |
| Walnuts | Oregano |
| Cauliflower | Mustard seeds |
| Cabbage | Romaine lettuce |
| Broccoli | Brussels sprouts |
| Winter squash | Summer squash |
| Collard greens | Spinach |
| Kale | Turnip greens |
| Strawberries | Green beans |
| Cloves | Pumpkin seeds |

## *DHA*

In recent years, scientists have begun to realize that the omega-3 fatty acid DHA is helpful to us at both the earliest and latest stages of our lives. For instance, a number of studies have shown that higher intakes of DHA significantly reduce the incidence of Alzheimer's disease and improve quality of life and memory in those affected by dementia. And in 2005, a review of more than fifty studies, published in the *American Journal of Clinical Nutrition,* concluded that higher DHA in babies' diets translates into better brain function, especially for cognitive and visual function. This is important to know because in the human infant, brain development undergoes its most rapid and complex growth during the last trimester of pregnancy and the first two years after birth.

During pregnancy, the mother supplies the baby with DHA, and she continues to supply it to the baby through her breast milk (or through infant formula fortified with DHA). DHA is the most abundant fat in the brain, accumulating in vast amounts during infant development and the first years of life. Interestingly, a 2000 study sponsored by the U.S. National Institute of Child Health and Human Development showed that adding DHA and AA (arachidonic acid, also known as ARA, an omega-6 fatty acid) to infant formula significantly boosted children's average intelligence. A control group received formula with no additives, a second group received formula with DHA added, and a third group received formula with DHA and AA. At eighteen months old, the children were given a Mental Development Index test that measures young children's memory, ability to solve simple problems, and language capabilities. The control group received an average score of 98—slightly below the national average of U.S. children. The average score for the DHA group was 102.4, and the DHA plus AA group received an average score of 105.

### *Omega-6*

In February of 2009, the American Heart Association stated that omega-6 fatty acids are a beneficial part of a healthy eating plan, and they recommended that people aim for at least 5 to 10 percent of their calories from omega-6 fatty acids. They also said that most Americans already get enough omega-6 in foods they are currently eating, such as nuts, cooking oils, and salad dressings. Omega-6s are beneficial to your overall health and may help in the prevention and/or treatment of the following conditions:

- Diabetic neuropathy

- Rheumatoid arthritis

- PMS

- Eczema

- Psoriasis

Some of the best food sources of omega-6s include:

| | |
|---|---|
| Pine nuts | Pistachio nuts |
| Sunflower seeds | Olive oil |
| Safflower oil | Grapeseed oil |

| Vegetable oil | Wheat germ oil |
| Corn oil | Walnut oil |
| Cottonseed oil | Soybean oil |

### The Omega Balancing Act

In an ideally healthy world, everyone would eat an equal amount of omega-3s and 6s, meaning there would be a ratio of 1:1. A balance of these two EFAs is necessary for optimal health. However, we don't live in an ideal (or balanced) world. These days, most Americans consume many more omega-6s than 3s, usually in ratios between 10:1 and 25:1. In our less-than-ideal world of processed and refined foods, full of vegetable and corn oils, there is a definite overabundance of omega-6s. This can cause serious health problems, including hyperactivity (ADD and ADHD), depression, and especially heart disease. If you want to achieve a healthy balance of omegas for you and your family, minimize the use of oils rich in omega-6 fatty acids, which may mean reducing your (and your children's) consumption of margarine, salad dressings, mayonnaise, and most fast and processed foods. At the same time, increase your consumption of omega-3-rich foods like cold-water fatty fish.

### The Question of Mercury

Both the Food and Drug Administration (FDA) and the Environmental Protection Agency (EPA) warn young children, women who might become pregnant, and those who are pregnant or nursing to completely avoid certain fish with high levels of mercury and other environmental contaminants. These fish include tuna, shark, swordfish, tilefish, and king mackerel. To get the latest updates on fish that are high in mercury or other toxins, you can visit the EPA Web site (www .epa/gov/mercury/fish/htm), the Environmental Defense Fund (www .edf.org), and the Marine Stewardship Council (www.msc.org).

## THE CHOLESTEROL CONUNDRUM

Research has shown that omega-3 oils, found largely in cold-water or deep-ocean fish, are particularly helpful in reducing the risk of heart disease. One of the reasons for this is that EFAs are cholesterol carriers; that is, they help move bad cholesterol (LDL) out of the body. If there is not enough EFA in the body, the cholesterol becomes attached to fat molecules, which usually end up coating arterial walls (thereby increasing the risk of heart disease).

We have been taught over the past few decades that foods such as fats, red meat, and especially eggs contain cholesterol and therefore should be avoided. But the latest data show that, once again, we have been throwing the baby out with the bath water.

Cholesterol, like fat, is essential to our survival. It helps produce vitamin D and helps the body repair damaged cell membranes. It is used as a building block of estrogen and testosterone, and it is necessary for the production of cortisone. Approximately 80 percent of the cholesterol in our bodies is produced by the cells themselves. Cholesterol is divided into "good" and "bad." Good cholesterol is high-density lipoprotein (HDL), which is carried to the liver, where it is broken down into bile and eventually eliminated from the body. Bad cholesterol is low-density lipoprotein (LDL), which carries fat and cholesterol throughout the body and deposits them in various spots, including the arteries.

**These are synthetic oils that the body attempts to utilize to regulate growth, to build healthy brain tissue. But it's substandard material.**

If you don't have enough cholesterol in your body, your cells will produce more or will grab some floating by in the bloodstream. If you greatly reduce the amount of cholesterol you're ingesting, the body will only produce more. So the warnings we have been given about eating cholesterol don't seem to hold true; eating foods that contain cholesterol doesn't, in fact, add much cholesterol to our bloodstream.

Saturated fat, however, has been shown to raise blood cholesterol. In fact, the cholesterol we get from our food has much less effect on the level of cholesterol in our blood than the amount of saturated fat we eat.

Margarine contains no cholesterol, which is why it was created in the first place, but it does contain the artificially saturated trans fatty acids. Therefore, margarine is probably more of a hazard to your heart than butter, even though butter contains cholesterol.

This is also where insulin enters into the equation. When you eat a high–saturated fat, high-carbohydrate, high-sugar diet, you increase the level of insulin in the body. Insulin signals the cells to produce more cholesterol. When the body produces more cholesterol, there is no need for cells to grab the excess floating by in the bloodstream. That excess is then free to build up where you don't want it, specifically in the arteries. If you decrease the amount of high-carbohydrate, high-sugar foods in your diet, you automatically reduce the level of insulin, and therefore the level of excess cholesterol, in your body. This is yet one more reason to monitor your family's diet so that it includes more high-quality good fats and fewer bad fats, carbs, and sugar.

## WHY THE BAD FATS ARE BAD FOR YOU

As with most things in life, even some of the "bad" fats are not all bad. Saturated fats, which have gotten such a bad reputation over the years, actually provide our bodies with a good source of energy when we are low on fuel, serve as shock absorbers for our internal organs, and insulate us against the cold. Fats also help to keep cell membranes fluid so that, for example, red blood cells can squeeze through capillaries. Like every other food that's been discussed in this book, saturated fats are harmful only when they are consumed in excess. It's not the saturated fat in a small amount of butter that's going to do us in; it's the great gobs of it that we spread on bagels, muffins, and pancakes. It's not the steak with a small amount of fat in it that's harmful; it's the deep-fried foods. It's all the cakes, cookies, cereals, and baked goods that are made with highly saturated palm and coconut oil or partially hydrogenated vegetable oil.

Hydrogenated oils are oils to which hydrogen has been artificially added at extremely high temperatures to solidify them and give them longer shelf lives. Overconsumption of hydrogenated oils can cause a child to be vulnerable to recurrent infections, inflammatory conditions, and learning disorders. These are synthetic oils that the body attempts to utilize to regulate growth, to build healthy brain tissue. But it's substandard material. The body is using a kind of fat that is not designed for the generation of healthy tissue. In addition, while some fats, like omega-3 fatty acids, are anti-inflammatory, hydrogenated oils tend to promote inflammation.

Margarine is probably the best known partially hydrogenated product. Although it was created to be a healthier alternative to the saturated fat found in butter, margarine unfortunately turned out to be an unhealthy alternative. The process of hydrogenating the fat causes it to change its molecular structure into trans fatty acid. Trans fatty acid stays in the bloodstream for a much longer period of time than other fats, and has a harmful effect on cholesterol levels—it lowers the level of good HDL cholesterol while raising the level of bad LDL cholesterol.

Both trans fats and hydrogenated fats can actually interfere with the body's ability to metabolize the good fats. Imagine that a cell membrane is like a popular night club, velvet rope and all. Fats, both good and bad, travel through the bloodstream and get in line to enter the club. Unfortunately, the gatekeepers can't really tell the difference between the good guys and the bad guys. If the club gets filled to capacity with bad fats, the good ones can't get past the ropes. That means that the bad fats are free to wreak havoc in the club, while the good guys and their helpful nutrients are not able to do their jobs.

You can avoid trans fats by staying away from fast foods and by reading the labels of packaged goods. Anything that contains hydrogenated oil or partially hydrogenated oil contains trans fats. Although there are many foods on the market now that say "0 trans fats" on the label, you won't be able to eliminate them completely as they are still in a huge number of foods on the shelves and on restaurant menus. And don't be fooled by protein bars and fat-free ice cream; they may contain trans fats as well. Remember the moderation mantra: You don't have to be fanatic about the evils of trans fats. Just try to keep the proportion of EFAs and unsaturated fats higher than the trans fatty acids.

## The "Is Butter Better?" Debate

If you browse the dairy aisle in any supermarket, you will find what seems like hundreds of different brands of butter, margarine, and "I'm not butter or margarine but I'm trying to taste like them" spreads. How do you know which is best for your health? It's a tough call. All of them derive 100 percent of their calories from fat. Butter has saturated fat, but it has no trans fat. Margarine has a good deal of trans fat but it also has unsaturated (good) fat. Check the label and choose a margarine with a total fat content of 3 grams or less. If you do choose margarine, look for a brand that contains phytosterols, natural plant compounds that have been shown to reduce LDL cholesterol by 6 to 15 percent when eaten in recommended amounts.

You might want to choose one of the butter substitutes or spreads such as Smart Balance or Country Crock Omega Light Plus or one of the many others like it on the market. These substitutes are made from vegetable oils and some do not have any trans fat or cholesterol. The best way to choose is by reading the label. Avoid any product that contains hydrogenated or partially hydrogenated oils to avoid trace amounts of trans fat. And then go by taste. None of these spreads really tastes like butter (even though they may claim otherwise). A petite pat of butter now and again won't do you any harm; eating any of these options by the spoonful is not a good idea. So choose the one that works best for your family and spread it around—in moderation.

## A LOW-FAT DIET FOR KIDS?

Our society has become obsessed with weight. There is good reason for this, up to a point. We can't ignore the obesity problem in this country. On the other hand, we can't let it be our only concern when dealing with how we feed our children.

Obviously, you want your child to gain weight as she grows. And during certain periods of growth, such as adolescence, it is normal for kids to store extra fat. That's when parents start to walk the difficult tightrope of knowing when a child has put on too much weight and when it's fat that he'll "grow out of." Some parents become so frightened of what they see as excess body weight, that they put their kids on restrictive and, in most cases, low-fat diets. Although it's good to be aware of too much fat in your child's diet, a low-fat or no-fat regimen can actually be harmful to their health.

**Sufficient fat must be included in the diet for children to support normal growth and development; therefore giving them low-fat and sugar-free products is a bad idea.**

We want to teach our children to have positive relationships with food. We don't want them to be scared of food or to feel like their whole lives revolve around what they're going to eat next, as that may be paving the way for future eating disorders like anorexia (see Chapter 13 for more about childhood obesity and eating disorders).

It's all about moderation. Should we monitor the amount of fat we're serving to our children? Of course. Should we teach them how to read labels and to learn to make healthier decisions about what they eat? Certainly. But we don't want them to feel that we're restricting their fat intake because they're fat (and therefore "bad" or "unlovable," which is how they're likely to interpret it). The focus should be on eating healthy.

If your children are overweight, it can be very tempting to put them on a no-fat or low-fat diet. But studies such as the one published in the *Nutrition Journal* in 2007 found that children burn substantially more fat than adults relative to their calorie intake. Researchers for this study also stated that sufficient fat must be included in the diet for children to support normal growth and development; therefore giving them low-fat and sugar-free products is a bad idea.

## What Is a Sufficient Amount of Fat?

How much fat is sufficient depends on how old you are. Up until about the age of two, children require 40 to 50 percent of their daily calories from fat. From two through the teen years, children require about 30 percent of their calories from fat. Moderately active adults require about 25 percent of their calories from fat. Most of the fats consumed should be unsaturated. If you want to keep track of the fats your kids are eating, keep a food log similar to the one in Chapter 4. Write down everything your child is eating and drinking for one whole day. Then check the labels and write down the number of calories and the number of grams of unsaturated, saturated, and trans fats. Add up the numbers (there are 4 calories per gram of protein and carbohydrate and 9 calories per gram of fat). You may have to approximate calories and fat grams for unlabeled foods, but you can find many of these numbers on the Internet. You don't have to be exact; you only want to get a general idea. Calculate the percentage of fat calories versus the number of total calories for the day. For instance, if your teen is eating 2,000 calories per day, approximately 600 of those calories (30 percent) should be coming from fats.

Also, add up the number of grams of each type of fat: unsaturated, saturated, and trans. If there are more saturated and trans fats than unsaturated fats, you may want to make some changes in your child's diet. The next time you shop, be sure to read food labels. If the ingredient list of a particular food includes hydrogenated or partially hydrogenated oil, it means the product is high in trans fats. Choose foods that are lower in saturated and trans fats, including lean meats, fish, and fresh fruits and vegetables.

### Optimizing Good Fats

Here are some more tips for optimizing good fats and keeping bad ones to a minimum:

- Have healthy snacks readily available. Keep sliced fruit in the refrigerator; make a dip using low-fat yogurt. And mix it up—if you have apples and bananas on hand one week, try mangoes and kiwi the next.

- Look for "saturated fat" information on food labels. If a product has 3 grams of fat or less per 100-calorie serving, it counts as a low-fat choice.

- Kids love spaghetti. Try whole grain or omega-3 enriched pasta, served with tomato sauce and a sprinkling of Parmesan cheese.

- If you're serving meat, choose lean cuts, which usually include the words "loin" or "round" in the name (e.g., sirloin, tenderloin, top round, ground round). Trim visible fat from the meat before cooking.

- You can lower fat counts by reducing the amount of frying you do. Choose baking, boiling, broiling, microwaving, poaching, roasting, or steaming instead.

## THE FAT BALANCING ACT

The same Goldilocks Principle we discussed in the chapter on wheat applies here as well. Too much fat is not good for your child, but neither is too little. That's why it's important to monitor how much fat—and what kind—your kids are consuming.

Children who don't get enough fat in their diet will definitely suffer the consequences. It will affect their mood and their immune system. It can affect their bowel function. They won't perform as well socially, and they won't have the physical stamina a child should have. It will affect their ability to focus and to think clearly. In the absence of the right amount of essential fatty acids, you will have a child who falls far short of his or her physical and mental potential.

On the other hand, children whose diets contain too much fat will show fewer outward symptoms besides just being overweight, but will suffer consequences nonetheless. They may end up with type 2 diabetes during their childhood years. Researchers are finding that many children and young adults are now showing signs of heart disease that had previously only been found in older adults. The ground is being set for disease later on in life. And, like children who lack fat in their diet, they will probably have less energy, perform poorly in school, and have a hard time managing moods.

Fats are a hot political topic these days as governments around the country are banning trans fats and requiring restaurants to post calories and ingredients. This is a good thing, as it helps us all be more aware of what we're actually eating. Teach your kids how to read these postings, and how to read food labels as well. You're never too young to build a healthy foundation for the rest of your life.

# Questions to Ask Your Child's Doctor

- Should children be tested for signs of heart disease or high cholesterol? If so, at what age?

- Should my child be taking omega-3 fish oil?

- Does a fat change depending on how I cook it?

- I didn't eat any fish during my pregnancy. I am currently nursing my baby—is it safe for me to eat fish now?

- What are the best fish to feed my children in order for them to get the omega-3 they need?

# Chapter 9 Take-Home Points

- Children need fat for their growth and development. But it's important that the fat, as much as possible, should come from healthy sources such as avocados and omega-3 fish oils.

- It's not fat in general that's causing us problems, it's that most of us are ingesting too much of the wrong kinds of fat and too little of the right kinds. The best thing we can do for ourselves and our kids is to learn to tell the difference.

- "Good" fats are those that are least saturated: omega-3s, omega-6s, monounsaturated, and polyunsaturated. The worst fats are the most saturated: hydrogenated, partially hydrogenated, and trans fats.

- The superstar fats are omega-3, omega-6, and DHA. Some of the best food sources of omega-3s are fatty fish, including mackerel, salmon, trout, tuna, herring, striped bass, sardines, and anchovies.

- In the human infant, brain development undergoes its most rapid and complex growth during the last trimester of pregnancy and the first two years after birth. Higher DHA in babies' diets translates into better brain function, especially for cognitive and visual function.

- If you want to achieve a healthy balance of omegas for you and your family, minimize the use of oils rich in omega-6 fatty acids, which may mean reducing consumption of margarine, salad dressings, mayonnaise, and most fast and processed foods. At the same time, increase your consumption of omega-3-rich foods like cold-water fatty fish.

- Avoid trans fats by staying away from fast foods and by reading the labels of packaged goods. Anything that contains hydrogenated oil or partially hydrogenated oil contains trans fats.

- Sufficient fat must be included in the diet for children to support normal growth and development; therefore giving them low-fat and sugar-free products is a bad idea.

Fats aren't the only substances that help or hinder the way the body functions. You may be surprised to know that there are billions of bacteria that reside in our intestines and contribute to the efficiency (or inefficiency) of the digestive system. They can have a tremendous impact on how well or ill your child feels. These bacteria are called probiotics, and they're essential to your child's health.

## Chapter 10

# Let's Get Specific: Probiotics

*When Isabella, a charming if somewhat pale three-year-old, first came into my office, she had deep dark circles under her eyes and she breathed with her mouth open. She was active but somewhat slow to respond to my playful questions. Her mother reported that she had had recurrent ear infections for which she had always been given antibiotics. At her last checkup, her regular pediatrician had recommended surgery to place tubes that would help drain the fluid in her ears.*

*Needless to say, Isabella's mother was not happy with the possibility of surgery for her young daughter. She brought her to my office for a second opinion. As I watched Isabella, I asked her mom a series of questions: Did she eat a lot of wheat and dairy? Yes. Did she snore? Yes. Did she have intermittent diarrhea? Yes. Did her tummy often appear bloated? Yes. Her mother also told me that Isabella often had large bulky stools that smelled much worse than her older brother's. She also said that Isabella frequently complained in the morning that her stomach hurt, but her doctor suspected that this was "school phobia."*

*When I examined Isabella, I found that her middle ears were full of fluid. Her turbinates (the glands inside the nose) were swollen, and she had lots of post-nasal drip. Her belly was soft but distended a bit and full of gas. She looked pale and exhausted.*

*I suggested that Isabella start on a new dietary regimen of daily probiotics and a decreased amount of wheat and dairy. Given that she had been on so many antibiotics, the probiotics helped enormously with her abdominal bloating and discomfort. Probiotics also helped to restore her intestinal immune system so that her intestinal tract was less reactive to food sensitivities and her respiratory tract produced less mucus in response. Her ear infections cleared up, she stopped complaining about stomachaches, the dark circles under her eyes disappeared, and she returned to being a cheerful, energetic three-year-old.*

*—From Dr. Geary's files*

The human intestinal tract is inhabited by thousands of strains of bacteria, some beneficial, some harmful. The balance between these strains can have a huge impact on how a person feels. Often, although your child may not be "sick," he may intermittently complain of a tummy ache, poor appetite, or appear more tired than usual. It may be that his intestinal tract is out of balance and his digestion is sluggish. It is worth considering the addition of probiotics to the diet.

Probiotics work by constantly adjusting the intestinal immune environment to help correct the balance between beneficial and harmful bacteria and help to prevent disease-causing bacteria from attaching to and colonizing the gut. They restrict the overgrowth of harmful bacteria and promote the growth of helpful bacteria, which in turn enhances digestion and absorption of nutrients.

## THE FRIENDLY BACTERIA

When a baby is floating around in the womb with nothing to do all day but grow and develop, its intestinal tract, from the mouth down to the end of the large intestine, is sterile. If you're looking for bacteria, those single-celled microscopic organisms we often think of as harmful and disease-producing, you won't find them in an unborn child's gut. Send that child through the birth canal, however, and before you can say "welcome to the world," bacteria begin to colonize throughout the intestinal system.

> **A Numbers Game**
>
> We're not talking small numbers here—the intestine alone contains up to 100 trillion bacteria, more than ten times the total number of cells in the entire body.

But don't let that worry you. The majority of these bacteria, also known as *gut flora,* are not only friendly but are, in fact, essential to our survival. Here are just some of the functions of our gut flora:

- Helps the intestinal system develop and function properly

- Assists in digestion and absorption of food and nutrients

- Breaks down dietary toxins

- Synthesizes vitamins

- Assists in the absorption of minerals

- Forms a natural defense barrier against harmful bacteria, toxins, and antigens that can cause disease or infection

But perhaps most important, gut flora has a significant impact on the immune system. It may come as a surprise to learn that about 80 percent of our immune cells actually live in our intestinal system. Because of that, our immune system is particularly vulnerable to our environment—everything we eat or drink is potentially laden with harmful microorganisms. In order to combat that potential harm and mount a healthy immune response, all mammals require beneficial bacteria. That's why it's so important to maintain a healthy balance of good bacteria versus bad, and that's where probiotics come into the picture.

## WHAT ARE PROBIOTICS?

Probiotic literally means "for life." The World Health Organization (WHO) defines probiotics as "live microorganisms, which when given in adequate amounts, confer a health benefit on the host." In other words, probiotics are living bacteria that are similar to the friendly bacteria found in the human intestinal system. They live symbiotically in the gut, meaning they form a give-and-take relationship where they help us fight off the bad guys in return for a warm place to live.

Most often, the bacteria come from two groups, *Lactobacillus* or *Bifidobacterium*. Within each group, there are different species (for example, *Lactobacillus acidophilus* and *Bifidobacterium bifidus),* and within each species, different strains or varieties (a few common probiotics, such as *Saccharomyces boulardii,* are yeasts, which are different from bacteria). Some of these probiotics are colonizing bacteria, which means that they are very "sticky" and adhere to the wall of the bowel. Others, like the species *bulgarica,* are transient; as *bulgarica* moves through the bowel it sweeps away some of the pathogens that may be harmful to us, and in its wake it leaves a healthier, pinker colon.

Probiotics are available in foods and in dietary supplements (e.g., capsules, tablets, and powders) and in some other forms as well (see our recommendations on page 151).

Interest in probiotics in general has been growing rapidly: Americans' spending on probiotic supplements, for example, nearly tripled from 1994 to 2003, and nowadays you can't turn on the television for more than five minutes without coming across a commercial for various probiotic-filled yogurts.

Although most fermented foods contain probiotics, yogurt is by far the most common place to find them. Read the label of most yogurt containers and you will find a phrase such as "This product contains live and active cultures." These cultures are probiotics. Not all brands are equally fortified, however, so be sure to read the label. A few of our favorites include Stonyfield Farm, makers of YoBaby and YoKids (available in most supermarkets), and Bio-K (available in most health food stores).

## PROBIOTICS AND CHILDREN

Probiotics are particularly important for infants and young children because this is when their immune systems encounter things like microbes, foods, and allergens (substances that are capable of producing allergic reactions) for the first time. Certain probiotics may help keep immune responses from overreacting and becoming hypersensitive.

Infants are often first introduced to probiotics through colostrum, the breast milk that comes in during the first few days after birth (colostrum has a high concentration of substances that protect babies from infections). The breast milk that comes in after those first few days contains large quantities of complex starches that promote the growth of *Bifidobacteria,* a type of healthy bacteria, in the infant's digestive system. The beneficial bugs in breast milk allow the baby to quickly build up a strong gut flora, which gives it the best protection against diseases.

**If you introduce unhealthy bacteria as you age, it becomes more and more difficult to get back to a normal state. Adding probiotic foods and supplements helps the gastrointestinal tract maintain a healthy bacterial balance from the start.**

Our recommendation is that infants stay on breast milk or formula until they are one year old. However, it is okay to introduce yogurt in small amounts (approximately 2 ounces a day) starting at about nine months. As we said in Chapter 7, it is difficult for infants to digest cow's milk. That's why yogurt is so good for them—it's got all the benefits of dairy without the digestive issues cow's milk presents. And remember that good bacteria are introduced through breast-feeding, so the longer a mother can continue to breast-feed her baby the better. But it's important that you don't feel guilty if you don't or can't breast-feed for every meal. Breast-feeding even once a day has great benefits.

There are options for those who cannot or choose not to breast-feed their babies. Some infant formulas now add *Bifidobacterium lactis,* a probiotic similar to that found in breast milk. Why is it so important to be sure babies start life with these healthy bacteria? It turns out that once initially colonized by bacteria in infancy, your immune system learns to recognize and accept these microorganisms for the rest of your life. If you introduce unhealthy bacteria as you age, it becomes more and more difficult to get back to a normal state. Adding probiotic foods and supplements helps the gastrointestinal tract maintain a healthy bacterial balance from the start.

As children are weaned off breast milk, their need for probiotics continues. Here are some of the issues that probiotics can help alleviate in children:

### Gas and Bloating

- Does your newborn cry and cry and cry, more than most other babies? Does the baby seem to have frequent abdominal pain? Is she particularly fussy after eating? Does the infant seem more comfortable when he's carried upright? One of the most frequent complaints in any pediatrician's office is about gassy, bloated babies. These babies cry incessantly and inconsolably with no identifiable cause. In a 2007 study of eighty-three breast-fed infants, supplementation with probiotics improved gassy symptoms within one week of treatments, compared to simethicone, a gas reducer. In fact, after twenty-eight days the average crying times of the infants in the probiotic group had decreased by about 75 percent, compared to only 26 percent for the control group.

### Lactose Intolerance

- If you are lactose intolerant, you are deficient in the intestinal enzyme lactase, which is needed to digest the sugar found in milk. When you consume more lactose than there is lactase in the cells of the intestinal lining, the undigested lactose travels down the intestines where it ferments and causes symptoms such as gas, bloating, abdominal pain, and rashes on the skin. When probiotics are consumed either as a supplement or in food, they can create lactose activity in the gut, improve digestion, and alleviate symptoms.

> **Are Probiotics Safe?**
>
> If you are worried about the safety of probiotics, you should know that they have been studied in more than seventy clinical trials involving 4,000 children with no reported side effects.

## Diarrhea

- Probiotics have been shown to be the most beneficial in acute pediatric diarrhea. Several large controlled studies showed significant decrease in the duration of diarrhea in children who received probiotics as a supplement, in milk, or added to a rehydrating solution. Use of probiotics has shown a reduction in duration of diarrhea by seventeen to thirty hours.

## Diarrhea Caused by Antibiotics

- Antibiotics are used to kill off bad bacteria that may be causing the body harm. Unfortunately, they often kill off good bacteria in the gut at the same time. Antibiotics frequently cause diarrhea as well when they disturb the natural balance of bacteria in your gut, causing certain bacteria to multiply far beyond normal numbers. Antibiotic diarrhea affects one in five people receiving antibiotic therapy. Researchers are now beginning to advocate the use of probiotics to restore the gut flora during and after a course of antibiotics. Some probiotics are inhibited or inactivated by antibiotics, rendering the probiotics ineffective. However, Bio Gaia's *L. reuteri* Protectis has been found resistant to several commonly used antibiotics and has been shown to reduce the frequency and intensity of antibiotic-associated effects.

## Eczema

- Before 1960 approximately 3 percent of children born developed atopic dermatitis, or eczema, an inflammation of the skin that can cause itching, crusting, scaling, and/or blisters. The current rate of children who develop the condition is more than 15 percent. This may be due to the hygiene hypothesis, which says that the rising incidence of immune disorders such as allergy is due to modern society's reduced exposure to environmental, mainly harmless microorganisms. In other words, we're too clean. Because of reduced exposure to dirt, our immune system develops differently, resulting in an abnormal or heightened allergic response to normal environmental allergens.

> **Probiotics are essential as an everyday adjunct to good health, not just as a solution to health problems.**

- Perhaps one way to combat this situation is to use probiotics to shore up the gut flora. In a Finnish study, over 150 expectant mothers with a history of atopic dermatitis were given supplements of probiotics daily for several weeks before delivery. Breastfeeding mothers continued to receive the probiotics after delivery, or the children received oral supplements for six months. Those babies had half the atopic eczema of the control group.

### Weight Control
- This is an area that is still being researched, but a study published in January 2008 in the journal *Molecular Systems Biology* showed that probiotics given to mice changed how the mice metabolized bile acids, which are made by the liver and emulsify fats in the upper gut. This means that probiotics can change how much fat the body is able to absorb. This may turn out to be a useful tool in the fight against childhood obesity.

### RECOMMENDATIONS
If you type in "probiotics" on your favorite search engine, you will probably find hundreds, if not thousands, of brands on the market. Not only that, there are many different types of probiotics. The choices can be overwhelming. Where do you begin?

If you are considering giving your child probiotics, the first step you should take is to consult your physician or health professional. Although probiotics are remarkably safe, they are like any other medicine or supplement in that they may not be right for everyone.

When we do recommend probiotics to our patients and clients, there are several brands we consistently rely on, including:

- **BioGaia**—Available as Probiotic Drops designed to help infants who suffer from digestive discomfort including gas and bloating.

- **Culturelle**—Easy-to-swallow capsules that help improve digestion, reduce upset stomach, and help maintain regular bowel movements. Culturelle is also commonly given to help healthy bacteria thrive when one is on antibiotics.

- **Natren**—Natren Life Start is specifically designed for infants and toddlers, especially those who are formula-fed or are born by cesarean section (and so do not have the benefit of acquiring beneficial bacteria as they pass through the birth canal).

The most important thing to remember is that probiotics are essential as an everyday adjunct to good health, not just as a solution to health problems.

# Questions to Ask Your Child's Doctor

- My child frequently has an upset stomach. Could this be helped by probiotics?

- Does my child need probiotics if he is taking an antibiotic?

- Will probiotics shorten the course of diarrheal illness?

- How often should my daughter take probiotics? Every day? Or only when she has an upset stomach?

- Can my son get enough probiotics if he eats yogurt every day?

- Does frozen yogurt have probiotics?

- How do you know if you have enough good bacteria so you can stop the probiotics?

# Chapter 10 Take-Home Points

- The human intestinal tract is inhabited by thousands of strains of bacteria, some beneficial, some harmful. The balance between these strains can have a huge impact on whether a person feels well or ill.

- Probiotics work by constantly adjusting the intestinal immune environment to help correct the balance between beneficial and harmful bacteria and help prevent disease-causing bacteria from attaching to and colonizing the gut. They restrict the overgrowth of harmful bacteria and promote the growth of helpful bacteria, which in turn enhances digestion and absorption of nutrients.

- Eighty percent of our immune cells actually live in our intestinal system. Probiotics are living bacteria that are similar to the friendly bacteria found in the human intestinal system. They live symbiotically in the gut, where they help fight off harmful microorganisms in the foods and drinks that we ingest.

- Although most fermented foods contain probiotics, yogurt is by far the most common place to find them. Look for ones that contain live and active cultures.

- Infants are often first introduced to probiotics through colostrum, the breast milk that comes in during the first few days after birth. These probiotics allow the baby to quickly build up a strong gut flora, which gives it the best protection against diseases.

- Infants should stay on breast milk or formula until they are one year old.

- It is important that babies start life with these healthy bacteria because once initially colonized by bacteria in infancy, your immune system learns to recognize and accept these microorganisms for the rest of your life.

- The most important thing to remember is that probiotics are essential as an everyday adjunct to good health, not just as a solution to health problems.

It would be wonderful if our bodies were in balance all the time and we never had to worry about things like whether our kids' intestines were full of the healthy probiotics they need. But since we don't live in such a world, we need to be sure that our children are getting all the nutrients they require. In some cases, that may mean supplementing their diets with some of the extra vitamins and minerals you'll find described in the next chapter.

CHAPTER 11

# Supplementing Good Health:
# The Role of Nutraceuticals for Kids

In an ideal world, children would get all the vitamins and minerals they need by eating a variety of healthy foods. If our children all ate as well as they should and exercised as much as they should, perhaps they wouldn't need to take any supplements, or *nutraceuticals* as we like to call them. The best advice we can give is to offer your kids foods from the different food groups each day and prepare meals with nutrients that complement each other. That means eating fresh fruits, vegetables, lean meats, fish, whole grains, nuts, and legumes.

Unfortunately, children don't always eat the way we would like them to eat. Americans (adults and children alike) rarely get enough fruits and vegetables in their diets. A picky eater might not get all the vitamins, minerals, and other important nutrients he or she needs. Some kids eat healthy diets most of the time; most kids eat healthy foods some of the time; and a few children rarely eat anything healthy at all, gobbling down junk food instead (which most likely contains very little nutritional value—just unhealthy fats, sugar, and calories).

Obviously, a healthy diet is just as important for children as it is for adults. When a child doesn't eat enough healthy foods, both his physical and mental development are negatively affected. His ability to learn may suffer. Imagine sitting in school all day when you have no energy, you can't pay attention, and you're having difficulty socializing with other kids. And all because your brain and body are starving for good nutrition.

**Keep in mind that taking supplements isn't a cure-all or a substitute for a healthy diet.**

That being said, we are fortunate in this day and age that many categories of supplements are available for enhancing and improving our bodies' natural abilities. Kids who don't get all the nutrition they need from their diets can take supplements as a good way to ensure that they get enough vitamins and minerals, as long as you keep in mind that taking supplements isn't a cure-all or a substitute for a healthy diet.

---

### Teach Your Children Well

This is so important it's worth repeating. Supplements *never* replace good nutrition. It's not a Band-Aid for healthy eating. We don't want to teach our children that popping pills is better than eating well. The best strategy is always a well-thought-out nutritional plan.

---

## THE EVOLUTION OF NUTRACEUTICALS

According to the U.S. Food and Drug Administration (FDA), a nutraceutical (a term put together from two words: *nutritional* and *pharmaceutical*) is any substance that is a food or a part of a food that has medical or health benefits. Nutraceuticals help prevent and treat disease. They can be single nutrients like vitamin C (nutrients are the chemical elements that make up a food), or they can be combined, such as in a multiple vitamin or mineral supplement. A nutraceutical can also be a medicinally active food, such as garlic or flaxseed, or derived from a specific component of food, such as the omega-3 fish oil that comes from salmon and other cold-water fish.

Many of the nutraceuticals we use today are based on plants and plant extracts. This is definitely not a new phenomenon. People have been using plants for the treatment of illnesses and injuries since prehistoric times. The Iceman, discovered in the Alps in 1991 and estimated to be some 5,300 years old, carried a bag of medicinal herbs, believed to be used to treat the parasites found in his intestines.

Herbs have been used traditionally in every human culture. More than 5,000 years ago, the Sumerians described medicinal uses for plants such as laurel, caraway, and thyme. Ancient Egyptians of 1000 B.C. are known to have used garlic, castor oil, coriander, and mint; a Chinese herbal guide dating back to 2700 B.C. lists 365 medicinal plants and their uses; and more than 700 medicinal plants are listed in an Indian Ayurvedic herbal guide from the sixth century B.C.

The practice continues today. According to the World Health Organization (WHO), 80 percent of the world's population presently uses herbal medicine for some aspect of primary care. We do not recommend that nutraceuticals be used in place of traditional medical care. But we do suggest that they can be used to shore up your child's health and well-being in light of the poor quality and overconsumption of much of the food we eat.

### NUTRACEUTICALS FOR EVERYDAY MAINTENANCE

The nutraceuticals we list in this chapter are ones we believe are best designed to keep children's bodies working in top form. We don't expect your kids to take all of them. You never want to overmedicate your children with prescription drugs, vitamins, or any other kind of supplement. Read through the various descriptions, note which ones you think will be helpful to your children, and then discuss them with your pediatrician, nutritionist, or dietitian (especially if your children are taking any other prescription or over-the-counter medications).

---

### Dosages

We have purposely not listed dosages for the nutraceuticals we recommend because dosages can differ according to your child's age and/or weight. Read the manufacturer's label for dosage information, but remember, no matter what the manufacturer's label says, always base the dosage on your child's weight, not her age. You can have a 30-pound two-year-old or a 30-pound four-year-old. If the label does not give you the information you need, consult your pediatrician or health care provider. All medication for children should be based on their weight.

---

## PROBIOTICS

Probiotics are so important we felt it was important to include them here, even though we spent a whole chapter on them (see Chapter 10). The most important thing to remember is that probiotics are essential as an everyday adjunct to good health, not just as a solution to health problems.

- **BioGaia**—BioGaia contains the probiotics *L. reuteri,* which produces the antimicrobial substance reuterin, which inhibits the growth of several kinds of unhealthy bacteria. BioGaia is available as chewable tablets, straws, and as Probiotic Drops designed to help infants who suffer from digestive discomfort including gas and bloating. You can even get BioGaia chewing gum for oral health. Just as there are bad bacteria in the gut, there are bad bacteria in the mouth. *L. reuteri* Prodentis has a documented effect on balancing the oral flora and reducing the levels of bad bacteria associated with oral problems such as bleeding gums and tooth decay.

- **Culturelle for Kids**—Use Culturelle for kids to help improve digestion, reduce upset stomach, and help maintain regular bowel movements. Culturelle is also commonly given to help healthy bacteria thrive when one is on antibiotics. To use, simply empty entire contents of one packet into cool food or drink. Culturelle is completely tasteless and odorless, and is 100 percent dairy- and gluten-free.

- **Natren**—Natren Life Start is specifically designed for infants and toddlers, especially those who are formula-fed or are born by cesarean section (and so do not have the benefit of acquiring beneficial bacteria as they pass through the birth canal).

## OMEGA-3 FATTY ACID

One common deficiency in children's diets is a lack of omega-3 essential fatty acid (EFA). EFAs are essential for proper nervous system and brain function, which is very important during those long school days (see Chapter 9). EFAs are critical for proper growth in children, especially for neural development and maturation of sensory systems. Recent studies have also suggested that supplementation with high-dose EPA/DHA concentrates may improve behavior in children with attention deficit hyperactivity disorder (ADHD).

Docosahexaenoic acid (DHA) is a normal component of breast milk and is especially important for optimal brain and eye function. DHA is also important in the function and maintenance of the immune system, hormone regulation, and general health. Deficiency in DHA has been linked to dyslexia, aggressiveness, depression, reduced intelligence, manic depression, and more. We recommend that once a child is off breast milk or formula, you add a small amount of DHA (50 to 100 mg) to your child's orange juice, oatmeal, or other food until they're old enough to add fish to their diet. If you are breast-feeding, make sure that your own diet includes enough DHA, or that you are taking a fish oil supplement.

This essential fatty acid can be found in pumpkin seeds, oily cold ocean fish like salmon, tuna, halibut, and sardines, and in canola oil and flaxseed oil. It can also be taken as a dietary supplement if kids don't like the strong taste of oily fish or the other foods.

- **Dr. Ron's Ultra Pure Blue Ice Fermented Cod Liver Oil—** From ancient Rome to Scandinavia to the South Seas, traditional cultures considered fermented fish oils sacred foods essential to well-being. Blue Ice is available in capsules, unflavored liquid, or cinnamon-flavored liquid. This product is additive free, and contains vitamins A and D as well as the essential fatty acids EPA and DHA.

- **Dr. Fuhrman's DHA Purity—**This vegetable-derived formula was developed to maximize purity and freshness and is entirely vegan. That means there is no fishy taste or odor. This product comes in liquid form and you need take only a few drops a day, so it can be added to almost anything you drink or eat.

- **Carlson for Kids Chewable DHA—**A fun and tasty way to provide your children with the nourishing benefits of DHA omega-3 oil. Each orange-flavored chewable soft gel provides 100 mg of DHA. This product is regularly tested (using the Association of Analytical Communities (AOAC) international protocols) for freshness, potency, and purity by an independent, FDA-registered laboratory and has been determined to be fresh, fully potent, and free of detectable levels of mercury, cadmium, lead, PCBs, and twenty-eight other contaminants.

- **Neuromins DHA by Vitabase**—Fish oil is the most common source of the essential fatty acid DHA for dietary supplements; however, Neuromins DHA is a unique fish oil DHA supplement because of a special formulation process that extracts DHA from algae, the fish's actual source for its DHA. This high-quality brand of DHA supplement is chemical-, pollutant-, and toxin-free.

## VITAMIN D

For decades, experts have told us to stay out of the sun and if we do go outside, to wear hats and immediately slather ourselves with sunscreen. Lately, though, a different story has emerged, especially where children are concerned. It turns out that they are not getting enough sun. In fact, a whopping 70 percent of American children are not getting enough vitamin D.

Vitamin D is often called the "sunshine vitamin" because the human body only makes it when exposed to sunlight. No one is suggesting that you allow your kids to sunbathe on the beach for hours unprotected. We strongly recommend sunscreen for you and your children, but discuss with your pediatrician, based on where you live, how much time your child can be out in the sun without sunscreen.

Vitamin D is crucial for the absorption and metabolism of calcium and phosphorous, which have various functions, especially the maintenance of healthy bones. Vitamin D is an immune system regulator; it has a key role in maintaining cognitive function; it can help reduce the severity and frequency of asthma symptoms; and it has been shown to help lower the risk of certain cancers.

Children with low levels of vitamin D tend to have higher blood pressure and lower levels of good cholesterol than their peers, and they have an increased risk of developing heart disease later in life. Those most at risk for vitamin D deficiency are darker-skinned children, particularly African-Americans and Hispanics, because their skin contains more melanin than lighter-skinned children, and melanin may prevent the skin from absorbing the sunlight it needs.

The American Academy of Pediatrics recommends that:

- Breast-fed and partially breast-fed infants should be supplemented with 400 IU a day of vitamin D beginning in the first few days of life.

- All non-breast-fed infants, as well as older children, who are consuming less than one quart per day of vitamin D-fortified formula or milk, should receive a vitamin D supplement of 400 IU per day.

- Adolescents who do not obtain 400 IU of vitamin D per day through foods should receive a supplement containing that amount.

Foods that contain vitamin D include salmon, canned tuna, egg yolks, beef or calf liver, cheese, and fortified sources such as milk, yogurt, and cereals; however, it is almost impossible to get enough vitamin D from diet. That's why you need to give your children vitamin D supplements, such as:

- **ChildLife Essentials Vitamin D3 Mixed Berry Flavor (ages six months and up)**—ChildLife Vitamin D3 is made especially for infants and children. Alcohol-free, all natural ingredients, optimum absorption, and natural berry flavor.

- **Carlson Labs Baby D Drops (ages newborn and up)**—This product is sugar-free, soy-free, corn-free, wheat-free, gluten-free, and preservative-free. For infants less than two years old, place one drop onto a pacifier or mother's nipple and allow the baby to suck for at least thirty seconds. For children over two years of age, it may be put on food, mixed in a drink, or taken from a spoon.

## MULTIVITAMINS

Although there are some high-quality multivitamins for children on the market, many contain sugar and/or poorly absorbed nutrients that are peed right out of kids' systems. Choose multivitamins designed specifically for children. Look for products with no artificial dyes or coloring and no artificial sweeteners. Follow the recommended dose, and remember that virtually all children's multivitamins contain flavors to make them enjoyable for children to take, and many come in cartoon shapes with bright colors. Make sure your child understands that they are not candy and shouldn't be taken more often than the label recommends. If you give your child vitamins that are in the form of gummies, they need to brush their teeth afterward because pediatric dentists are now reporting that gummies are a significant source of cavities. If the multivitamin contains an adequate dosage of vitamin D, there is no need to give your child any additional vitamin D. Here are a few multivitamins we recommend:

- **Thorne Research Children's Basic Nutrients**—These contain the most bioavailable nutrients, in small, easy-to-swallow, kid-size capsules. The two-part capsule may also be taken apart and the contents emptied into food or liquid.

- **Dr. Sears Little Champions Children's Multivitamins (for ages two and up)**—These natural fruit-based soft chews serve as an ideal nutrient delivery system for children and taste good as well. They contain no artificial color, artificial flavors, or high-fructose corn syrup.

## ADJUNCT SUPPLEMENTS FOR SPECIFIC PURPOSES

When your child's diet is not able to meet all the nutrient needs of his or her body, supplements may be useful to help treat specific problems.

These are not supplements that need to be taken every day; rather they are to be used only when a specific problem arises. As long as your child is eating a relatively balanced diet, there is no need for her to be taking a dozen different pills or liquids. Should you decide (after consulting with your health professional) to give your child supplements, here are some suggestions.

### Iron Deficiency

Iron is necessary for the body to make hemoglobin, the oxygen-carrying component of red blood cells. It's important for young children and teens to get enough iron in their daily diets. Infants who are breast-fed get enough iron from their mother; infants who are not breast-fed should get iron-fortified formula. Iron levels naturally decline as they get older, whether they're breast- or formula-fed, but much more so if they're breast-fed, which is why, after six months of age babies should be fed iron-fortified cereal.

Some children are at risk for iron deficiency. Toddlers who may not be eating enough iron-containing or iron-fortified foods are at risk. Teen girls are at risk if their diets don't contain enough iron to counteract the loss of iron during menstrual bleeding. And teen athletes may lose iron through sweating during intense exercise.

There are a number of iron-rich foods that should be a part of your child's diet so that iron deficiency does not occur, including:

- Salmon
- Dark poultry
- Tuna
- Red meat
- Eggs
- Beans and peas
- Fruits

- Leafy green vegetables

- Blackstrap molasses

- Enriched grains

- Iron-fortified breakfast cereals

If your child is in one of the risk categories previously mentioned or is not getting enough dietary iron, it may be necessary to give him or her iron supplements.

---

### Too Much Iron Is NOT a Good Thing

It's extremely important to remember that your child should not be given potent iron supplements without first consulting a doctor. Taking too much iron can cause constipation and can also cause serious poisoning in children.

---

Iron is best absorbed when taken with food because it can occasionally cause stomach upset. Iron should not, however, be given with milk or caffeinated beverages, which will interfere with absorption. Vitamin C enhances iron absorption, so try to include plenty of sources of vitamin C in your child's diet. If you do choose to give your child iron supplements, here are some suggestions:

- **Ferrous Sulfate Iron Supplement Drops by Rx Choice**—These drops should be given immediately after meals and may be given directly into the mouth or mixed with water or fruit juice.

- **Enfamil Fer-In-Sol Iron Supplement Drops (for infants and toddlers)**—Scientifically formulated to meet a child's supplementary iron needs. Use only as directed by your child's doctor.

## *Lactoferrin*

Lactoferrin comes from the word *lacto,* meaning milk, and the word *ferrin,* meaning iron. Lactoferrin is found naturally in the body in breast milk, tears, and other body fluids. It's the first line of defense for any opening in the body. Lactoferrin binds and transports iron in the blood, making it beneficial for iron deficiency. It also provides numerous benefits to the immune system, and is a powerful prebiotic (a food source for probiotic bacteria, to make them more effective; some prebiotics have been shown to enhance the absorption of important minerals like calcium and iron). Lactoferrin is often provided through dairy foods; since we recommend limiting the amount of dairy your child consumes, lactoferrin can be considered an alternative to high-fat dairy products.

- **Lactoferrin Gold 1.8 by Nikken**—This product is lactose-free and is recommended for children over the age of four. It inhibits the growth of harmful bacteria, viruses, fungi, and parasites in the digestive system.

- **NutriCology Laktoferrin**—High-quality lactoferrin obtained from Netherlands or New Zealand range-grazed cattle; 95 percent purity and low iron content.

## HEALTHY IMMUNE SYSTEM

When your child eats a balanced diet, including a variety of fruits and vegetables, she is literally feeding her immune system. Since many children go through phases when they don't eat as well as they should, their immune systems are not always working at peak efficiency. In addition, they're often exposed to more germs and illnesses than adults because of their close proximity to other children at school. Every parent knows when a bug has hit the schoolyard—soon whole classrooms are sneezing and coughing and half the class is staying home. At these times it's especially important to keep your child's immune system well nourished and to give it a boost with a few powerful supplements.

### Vitamin C

We all know that vitamin C helps prevent colds, right? Not so fast. This theory was put out by scientist Linus Pauling in the early '70s, and for these many years, we have believed it. But recent studies have shown that vitamin C supplements do not make a cold shorter or less severe. Researchers found that the average adult who suffers with a cold for twelve days a year would still suffer for eleven days a year if he or she took a high dose of vitamin C every day during that year, and the average child who suffers about twenty-eight days of cold illness a year, would still suffer for twenty-four days after taking a year's worth of daily high-dose vitamin C. Other studies have produced different results, however, showing that vitamin C does cut the length of time that a cold lasts. Taking vitamin C beforehand does not seem to prevent people from catching a cold in the first place.

Does that mean you should get rid of this supplement? Not at all. Vitamin C has plenty of other benefits. It is a powerful antioxidant that neutralizes free radicals that can cause damage to cells and lead to problems such as inflammation and even cancer. In fact, adequate intake of vitamin C has been shown to be an immune system booster and is excellent for brain, eye, and hearing health. It also enhances iron absorption, promotes wound healing, helps build collagen (connective tissue between muscle and bone), and aids in the production of neurotransmitters.

Humans do not have the ability to make their own vitamin C; therefore, we must obtain it through our diet. Some good food sources of vitamin C are oranges; red, yellow, and green bell peppers; strawberries; kiwi; cantaloupe; brussels sprouts; sweet potatoes; and broccoli. If your child isn't getting enough vitamin C through food, we recommend the following supplements:

- **Amalaki by Morpheme**—This product is made from the Amla fruit, also known as the Indian Gooseberry. Amalaki is the most widely used herb in the Ayurvedic system of medicine. It has one of the richest concentrations of vitamin C of any edible plant on earth, and is a powerful antioxidant agent for boosting

immunity. It is free of yeast, gluten, wheat, corn, dairy products, or any other artificial additives.

- **Carlson for Kids Chewable Vitamin C**—Carlson for Kids
  Chewable Vitamin C provides 250 mg of vitamin C with calcium in a tasty chewable tablet. It is gentle to the teeth and in
  the stomach. It is sweetened with fructose and sorbitol, naturally occurring sweeteners in fruit.

## Zinc

Zinc is a mineral that is essential to good health, as it is involved in hundreds of chemical reactions that take place in the body. It is an important
contributor to a healthy immune system (it activates white blood cells to
fight infection), and it plays a critical role in growth and development.
It's particularly important for infants, children, and pregnant women to
get enough zinc. Zinc also helps add calcium to bones and teeth, lowers
blood sugar, and improves brain function.

Zinc deficiencies can lead to chronic fatigue, diarrhea, insulin resistance, and loss of taste or smell. It can make it more difficult for the
body to fight off infection and can cause night blindness, poor appetite,
poor memory, and possibly attention deficit disorder.

If your child eats a healthy diet, he probably gets enough zinc already.
The best food sources of zinc are red meat, hummus, wheat germ, wheat
bran, nuts, and seeds. Crabs, lobster, and oysters are also good sources
of zinc, but they're not exactly kid friendly. Cocoa powder, however, is
child friendly and is also a good source of zinc, so if your kids want a
sweet snack, a small square of dark chocolate is a delicious, nutritious
alternative. Vegetarians usually need more zinc supplementation than
meat eaters, since meat is high in bioavailable zinc and may enhance zinc
absorption. In addition, vegetarians typically eat high levels of legumes
and whole grains, which inhibit zinc's absorption. Poor dietary habits
such as excessive consumption of sugar or carbohydrates are also known
to reduce zinc absorption.

In the past several years, there have been a number of studies looking at the possible link between zinc and ADHD. Some studies suggest

that children with ADHD might have lower levels of zinc in their body than children without this disorder. Researchers have reportedly seen improvement in children with ADHD who took zinc along with traditional ADHD treatment. Several studies have shown zinc supplements can reduce hyperactivity and impulsivity. More research is needed in this area. Needless to say, if you're thinking of adding zinc supplements to your child's diet, this is something that must be discussed with your health professional.

Zinc, in the form of zinc gluconate glycine lozenges (which can be found in any drug store), can also be used to reduce the duration of the common cold. Of the 62 million common colds requiring medical attention in the United States each year, more than 80 percent affect school-age children. Treatment with zinc gluconate glycine lozenges has been shown to significantly decrease cold duration and antibiotic use in school-age subjects. So if your child comes down with a cold, zinc lozenges, which dissolve in the mouth, can shorten the number of days the cold will last.

The best way to give your children more zinc is to add zinc-rich foods to their diet. If you do go for zinc supplements, here are a few we recommend (check with your health care provider for use in children under the age of twelve):

- **Cold-EEZE**—Reduces the duration and symptoms of the common cold including cough, stuffy nose, sore throat, sneezing, post-nasal drip, and hoarseness. The Cold-EEZE proprietary (zinc gluconate glycine) formula is believed by researchers to interfere with the cold virus's (rhinovirus) ability to reproduce. Cold-EEZE uses natural flavors and has no preservatives or colors.

- **Life Extension Zinc Lozenges**—Zinc lozenges have become popular supplements to use when people feel a runny nose coming on. When zinc is sucked in the mouth in lozenge form, it binds to specific cell receptor sites in the nasal/oral cavity, which inhibits the ability of undesirable entities to take hold.

This product contains no milk, egg, fish, peanuts, crustacean shellfish (lobster, crab, shrimp), tree nuts, wheat, yeast, gluten, or rice. It contains no artificial sweeteners or flavors.

## METABOLISM

Metabolism, simply defined, is the sum total of all the biochemical processes that take place in the body. Every individual's metabolism functions at a different rate. Some people burn fuel (food) at a fast rate; others have a much slower rate. The thyroid and the hormones it releases control much of the body's metabolism. When the thyroid begins to malfunction or a disease affects its processes, the metabolism of the body can become seriously impacted. One of the biggest changes that can occur as a result of a thyroid problem is weight gain or weight loss.

The thyroid cannot function without iodine, a mineral that is found in iodized salt, seafood, and dark green vegetables such as kelp, kale, and spinach. Iodine is essential for the production of the thyroid hormones that regulate metabolism. Iodine deficiency is very common in many parts of the world. Although it is not so common in America due to the introduction of iodized salt in the 1920s, it is slowly creeping back up. That's because we are becoming a low-sodium society. Worried that salt was causing or contributing to high blood pressure in adults, many food manufacturers lowered the amount of salt in the foods they sell. Many high blood pressure–conscious parents have started using sea salt as a substitute for common table salt—but sea salt does not contain iodine. We are teaching our children that salt is something to be avoided.

Symptoms of iodine deficiency include low energy, dry skin, constipation, intolerance of cold temperatures, brittle nails, and thin hair. Children are particularly susceptible to iodine deficiency because food sources are mainly fish and sea vegetables, which are not high on a child's list of favorite foods, and iodized table salt. The reality is, however, that most kids eat enough junk food and commercially processed snacks to get plenty of salt in their diets.

The thyroid hormone is an essential part of brain development. If a child does not get enough iodine, their learning and cognition can be affected. Children require different amounts of iodine, depending on how old they are:

| | |
|---|---|
| Infants | 40 to 50 micrograms per day |
| Ages 1 to 3 | 70 micrograms |
| Ages 4 to 6 | 90 micrograms |
| Ages 7 to 10 | 20 micrograms |
| Ages 11 and up | 150 micrograms |

There can be complications associated with consuming too much iodine, so you should always check with your health professional to determine if supplementation is necessary. A good way to supplement iodine in the diet is the use of the following product:

- **Eden Organic Seaweed Gomasio.** Organic dry-roasted sesame seed ground with sea salt and the mineral-rich sea vegetables kombu, dulse, and nori. Replaces table salt. Sesame oil coats the salt and greatly reduces its harshness. This seasoning is a good way to get iodine from seaweed in children, who probably won't eat seaweed in its natural state.

# Questions to Ask Your Child's Doctor

- Does my child's diet seem well-balanced?

- Are there any specific tests you would recommend to check if my child's nutritional status is good?

- My child is a picky eater; does she need vitamins?

- Should I increase my child's supplements when we travel, since he eats nothing but junk food when we're on the road?

- I want to give my child omega-3 supplements, but she refuses to take them. What should I do?

- Is there a brand of supplements that you particularly recommend?

- Which three supplements would you rank as most important for my child at her age?

- Eating is already a battle with my child. Should I waste more energy fighting over supplements?

# Chapter 11 Take-Home Points

We recommend the following nutraceuticals for children (always check with your health professional first):

**Everyday Maintenance**
- Probiotics

- Omega-3

- Vitamin D

- Multivitamin

**Adjunct Supplements for Specific Purposes:**
- Iron

- Lactoferrin

- Vitamin C

- Zinc

- Iodine

The chapters in this section of the book have helped you understand the relationship between the immune system and the foods children eat. The next section will help you and your child understand the connection between good nutrition, good health, and living in the real world.

# PART III

## LIVING (AND EATING) IN THE REAL WORLD

Throughout this book, we've repeatedly said that you don't have to eliminate entire food groups from your child's diet, that you don't have to be the food police, that you don't want your child to be that "freaky kid" who can't eat anything at a party or a playdate.

That being said, you do have a certain amount of responsibility to keep your children healthy. You may not be the food police, but you are the food provider. Just as you need to teach your children right from wrong, you also need to teach them healthy from unhealthy. That means you need to educate yourself about your child's nutritional needs, and you need to help your child understand that there are consequences to eating foods that are bad for him and benefits to eating foods that are good for him.

### Take Charge of Your Kids

*A couple came into my office with their eight-year-old son. He had been diagnosed with ADHD. He was taking Adderall and Ritalin and a sleeping pill at night. He was constantly anxious, irritable, and moody. His parents didn't know what else to do. After hearing his history, I asked the parents what his diet was like. "His diet?" said his mother. "He's not on a diet." "I don't mean a weight loss diet," I said. "I mean what does he usually eat?" I was surprised to hear that what he usually ate was a combination of fast food meals, mac and cheese, and candy snacks throughout the day. His parents did not eat this way at all. They knew his eating habits were not nutritionally sound, yet they were unwilling to set boundaries for their child. They didn't want to upset him or cause a confrontation. It took several visits before I was able to convince them that all the medication in the world would not help him if he continued his sugar and fat-filled way of eating. His parents finally realized they needed to set some nutritional rules for their son. They slowly cut back on his fast food meals and especially his candy snacks during the day, for which they substituted yogurt, fruit, and carrot sticks. Within a month his behavior had improved significantly and within six months they were able to cut back on his medicine.*

*—From Oz Garcia's files*

You are the shaper of your kids' lives. If you don't do it, some other outside influences will be shaping them for you. In the next few chapters, you'll learn how to talk to your children about food and help them understand that making healthy choices is part of growing up. It's not always easy to eat well in the real world. Teach them while they're young and it will stay with them through the rest of their healthy lives.

# CHAPTER 12

# How to Talk to Kids About Food: Stopping Problems Before They Start

A family of four is sitting around the dinner table. Well, Mom isn't actually sitting. She's running back and forth from table to stove to refrigerator. Little Suzy has refused to eat her peas—in fact, she's refused to eat anything at all—so Mom is busy pleading with her to take "just one bite" while heating up canned corn because she knows it's something Suzy is more likely to eat. Big brother Nathan has decided he doesn't like the turkey burgers Mom has made for dinner, so now she is making him a peanut butter and jelly sandwich, the only thing he wants to eat these days. And Dad, oblivious to it all, looks up from his Blackberry and asks, "Honey, where's that barbeque sauce you know I like?"

Unfortunately, this scenario is all too typical in American homes these days. Even when a family does sit down to a meal together, they seem to be leading separate lives, with the frazzled Mom or Dad trying to please everyone and maybe even squeeze a little healthy eating in at the same time. It often seems like an impossible task. Kids are influenced by so many external stimuli when it comes to food: TV commercials for candy and junk foods of all kinds, friends who seem to subsist on fries and chips, sugary treats they get at parties and playdates. Well-meaning parents are encouraged to disguise healthy foods by sneaking them into sweet treats or by making food into funny faces on the plate, rather than finding ways to help kids understand the role good nutrition has in their lives.

> Even when a family does sit down to a meal together, they seem to be leading separate lives, with the frazzled Mom or Dad trying to please everyone and maybe even squeeze a little healthy eating in at the same time. It often seems like an impossible task.

The reality is that there is a lot we can do nutritionally to keep kids healthy. It's part of our job as parents, because how we feed our kids now and how we talk to them about what they eat has a huge impact on our children's lifelong relationship with food.

## A Continual Conversation About Food

Taking on the responsibility of being family nutritionist is difficult for every parent. How can you compete with a silly rabbit who thinks a certain sugary cereal is so good, he tries to steal it away from kids? What can you do when you take your kids shopping and stores purposely put kid-friendly foods on lower shelves so children can grab them and stuff them into the grocery cart before you even know it? Why would a child want the fish and broccoli he's being served at home when the television tells him he can go to a fast food restaurant and get a box full of tasty treats—and a plastic toy to boot!

Teaching your children about health and nutrition may seem like a daunting task. But the sooner you start, the easier it will get. Teach your kids to be detectives to uncover what's really in the packaged foods they want to eat, and you give them a head start on making better food choices as they get older.

### But I Want It!

What do you do when your child starts the old whining routine of "But I want it!" when it's something you'd rather they didn't eat? Start a conversation. Here's one scenario: You're walking through the grocery store with your six-year-old, Jordan. He picks up a box of his favorite cereal and tosses it in the cart. You tell him that you'd like him to try a healthier cereal instead.

"But why?" asks Jordan. "This is healthy. It's got berries in it." You show him the box and explain that there aren't any real berries in the box, and that this cereal's main ingredient is sugar. "But I want it!" says Jordan. "The commercial says it's good for you."

You explain that commercials don't always tell the whole story, and that you want him to eat foods that are truly good for him and will help him grow up to be strong and healthy. You may not convince him on this trip. He may be angry or sulk. But you can continue the conversation another time. The most important thing is that you start talking about how food works to give you energy and keep your body growing properly and that certain ingredients are better for you than others. Let your children know that the reason you're being careful about what they eat is because of how much you care about them.

Here are some suggestions on helping your kids make healthy choices:

- Watch commercials with your kids and talk about them afterward. Ask your children if they believe everything they heard, and find out why or why not. Explain that directors use tricks to make food look more appealing, and that they are most interested in selling the product, not in keeping your family healthy.

- Try not to make food the enemy. Let them know that some foods are for once-in-a-while treats, while others are for every-day nutrition. You don't want to scare them into thinking that they are being terribly bad if they eat something that is normally off limits.

- Don't try to change everything at once. Introduce one new food at a time, and wait a while before you introduce another one. If your kids are used to eating fast foods and candy, slowly reduce the amount or the number of times you go to the drive-through. Major changes are often scary for kids.

## A FAMILY AFFAIR

There is no getting around it: Sitting down to a family meal with everyone present at the same time seems more like a nostalgic scene out of a '50s sitcom than a possibility in twenty-first-century real life. It may not be achievable on a daily basis, especially as children get older. But study after study tells us that it is well worth the effort—both psychologically and nutritionally.

One study conducted by the University of Minnesota showed that the more meals families ate together, the less teens smoked cigarettes or marijuana or drank alcohol; they had higher grade point averages and fewer symptoms of depression. And a Harvard University study showed that families who ate meals together almost every day ate more healthfully, consuming higher amounts of calcium, fiber, vitamins B6, B12, C, and E, and consuming less fat than families who ate together less frequently.

When you prepare meals at home, you have more control over the foods your children are eating (at least once a day). Plus, children tend to mimic their parents' values and attitudes. When you make family mealtime a priority, it will become more of a priority to your kids as well. If they see that you put in the time and effort to plan and prepare the family meal, they are more likely to see healthy eating as important.

> When you make family mealtime a priority, it will become more of a priority to your kids as well. If they see that you put in the time and effort to plan and prepare the family meal, they are more likely to see healthy eating as important.

When you sit down to eat, get rid of as many distractions as possible. Let the phone calls go to voice mail. Turn off the radio and TV, put down the electronics and the video games. Learn to listen to each other.

Family mealtime should be a positive experience. It may be a good time to go over what happened in school today, but it's not the time to lecture your kids on how disappointing their test grades have been or to express your disapproval for the way they behaved at grandma's house last weekend. You don't want your kids to associate mealtimes with stress or criticism, and you don't want them to slam their utensils on the table, stop eating, and rush from the table in a fit of anger. Mealtime is for stimulating positive conversation and sharing ideas. It should be a calm, casual affair.

If you can keep family mealtime to a set schedule, that's great. That's not always possible or practical, however, so you may have to mix it up a bit. If you can't all eat together at dinner, see if you can all make it to breakfast at the same time. Pack a picnic lunch and meet at the ball field before a game. Where and when you have the meal isn't as important as simply spending time all together enjoying a few nutritious dishes.

### Get Your Children Involved

One way to encourage your children to look forward to family meals is to get them involved in the planning and preparation. Talk to them about the various components that go into a balanced meal, and allow them to make choices in each category. For instance, you might say, "We need a carbohydrate as a side dish at dinner. Which would you like to help me prepare, rice or sweet potatoes?" If they're too young to grasp the concept of carbs, just say, "Let's make something good to go with the chicken," then give them a choice of what to cook.

Even young children can help prepare foods that don't require knives or other dangerous kitchen utensils. They can tear up lettuce for a salad, stir things in bowls, pour premeasured ingredients into baking dishes, or set the table. Older kids often enjoy getting to use food preparation equipment like salad spinners. Another fun way to get kids involved, and to teach them responsibility, is to ask them to take charge of creating and preparing a meal themselves once a month or so.

If your children are shopping with you, teach them how to read labels. Ask them to pick out the brand with the least amount of saturated fat, or to compare amounts of sodium. This not only helps you prepare healthy meals, but it also gets them thinking about what they're eating at home, at school, and at their friends' homes.

Though it's not always possible (depending on where you live), kids also get excited when they can help you grow their own vegetables in a backyard garden, participating in the process from planting to harvesting to preparation. This often makes them more likely to try new foods.

## HOW (NOT) TO FIGHT THE FOOD BATTLE

*A few months before Amelia turned two, she started refusing to eat dinner. It didn't seem to matter what her mother served—whatever it was, Amelia was more likely to throw it on the floor than to put it in her mouth. She ate breakfast and she usually ate lunch, but dinner soon became an all-out war between Amelia and her mom. When her mother brought her to my office, she was visibly agitated while she spoke to me, with Amelia in the room, about Amelia's upsetting dinnertime behavior. "I've tried everything," her mother said. "I've tried sitting her in front of a video during mealtime. I've tried making stupid airplane sounds. My husband invented a 'dinner dance' that makes her laugh so I can try to sneak food into her open mouth. I've made her meals into clowns and smiley faces. Nothing I do seems to work. I am so worried that she is not getting the nutrients she needs. I'm afraid she'll waste away to nothing."*

*Looking at the perfectly plump two-year-old in front of me, now as agitated as her mother, I assured Mom that Amelia was not going to starve herself—children do not let themselves starve—and that she was going through a normal stage of wanting to assert her control and using food as the means to do it. I gave her mother a tip-sheet about managing mealtime (see below) and advised her to relax about her daughter's eating habits. The more she stressed out about it, the more her daughter would figure out how to manipulate Mommy into getting her way.*

*—From Dr. Geary's files*

In most cases, there is no need to be so worried that kids are not meeting their nutritional needs. Studies have shown that if you look at what a child eats in a day or even over one week, you'll probably find it's top-heavy with one food category or another. But if you look at it over a month, you'll find a pretty balanced diet. In other words, they might not eat healthy within one twenty-four-hour period, but over the course of a month it will all balance out.

The most important thing to remember is that kids don't starve themselves. When they get hungry enough, they'll eat. The more you make a big deal out of it, the more stubbornly they will stick to their "I'm not going to eat anything just to spite you" attitude. You've always got to pick your battles with kids, and food should not be one of them. You will lose every time.

So how do you handle those dinnertime disputes? Here's our advice for managing mealtime:

- Establish a routine and stick to it as best you can. It can be difficult on special occasions or if you're traveling, but kids often thrive on structure.

- Serve your child a dinner that contains three items (preferably the same three items you're eating for dinner); for example, chicken, rice, and carrots.

- If your child eats all his carrots and wants more (and is eating only the carrots and nothing else), go with it. Give him more carrots. Don't force him to eat the chicken or the rice—and most important, don't go make him a hamburger because he won't eat the chicken. Explain the rule: If you want more of something that's on your plate, you can have it. If you don't want anything, you don't get another choice. Eat what you're served or eat nothing (remember, he won't starve).

- If he comes to you an hour later and says "I'm hungry," he can eat what he didn't eat earlier. But he doesn't get a different menu of foods.

- Don't insist that your child join the clean plate club. Sometimes she will be hungrier than at other times. If she says she's full or pushes her food away, respect her feelings and clear her plate away. You don't want to teach your children to keep eating even after they feel full.

- No negotiation allowed. No bribes. No "food as reward" tactics. Who amongst us hasn't said, at one time or another, "Two more bites and you can have ice cream for dessert," "Eat your spinach and you'll get a cookie," or "Clean your plate and you can have a candy after dinner"? It may get them to take a few more bites, but it will also convey the message that healthy food is something they have to "get through" before they can enjoy the more valuable treats they've been promised.

- No threats allowed. The other side of meal negotiation is to say, "If you don't eat your chicken you're going right to bed with no TV and no video games." It doesn't help to yell and scream, "If you don't eat this broccoli now, you will not have dinner and you will eat it cold for breakfast." Who would behave after that kind of threat? This not only cultivates negative relationships between your kids and food, it also fosters negative relationships between you and your kids.

## HOW TO KEEP A PICKY EATER HEALTHY

Some children will eat everything put in front of them, while others have a more selective palate. Some go through stages where they will eat only one food for days or even weeks at a time, or where they don't want one type of food to touch another. These developmental stages are normal. But what do you do when your child's meals are so limited that they lack variety and color? You may have tried all kinds of tricks, and still your child rejects almost everything he or she is served.

The truth is there are no tricks to getting kids to eat. If you're giving them healthy food and they don't eat it right away, don't push them. Eventually they will eat it because they're hungry. Just keep offering them the same healthy choices and before you know it, they will get hungry enough to put it in their mouths.

Research has shown that it can take between eight to ten tries before a child will accept a new food. Don't attempt to introduce new foods if your child is in a bad mood, is not hungry, or is overtired. The result will not be pleasant. Wait for a better time. Be sure your child sees you eating the new food as well; children love to imitate what adults around them do.

Here are some adjustments you can make to simple meals so that you know your child is getting as many nutrients as possible:

- **Pasta:** Many picky eaters rely solely on pasta for dinner and/or lunch, some with butter, some with cheese, and some with sauce. You can get a little more nutrition in them by swapping wheat-based pasta for pasta made of rice or quinoa. If you don't announce the change and continue to use their favorite sauces and toppings, they'll probably never notice the difference.

- **Snacks:** Whole-rye crackers with some cream cheese can be a healthy and plain snack, so can popping your own plain popcorn. Quinoa bars (which you can find in most health food stores or online) are delicious. You can also give them organic string cheese. Keep some dried fruit on hand for when you go out.

- **Drinks:** Limit high-calorie drinks, which fill them up before mealtimes. Stay away from juices as much as possible. They're high in calories and don't pack the nutrients and fiber of whole fruits. If your child won't drink plain water, try adding a slice of lemon or lime to give it flavor. If you do decide to give your child juice, pick a juice with the least amount of sugar and dilute it with 50 percent water. Look for juice that has calcium added as well.

- **Fruit:** If your child isn't a big fruit eater, try making her a smoothie. You can add a small amount of protein powder without changing the taste and texture, as well as some ground flaxseed for fiber and omega-3 oil for fat. Include low-calorie fortified fruit juice, yogurt, or frozen yogurt if you want to add some calcium.

## Feeding Your Kids on the Go

Getting kids from one place to another is difficult enough. Trying to feed them while traveling can be a nightmare. Careful planning helps. Here are some thoughts on how to navigate your child's nutritional needs during travel.

**If you are bringing snacks from home, remember:**

- For travel lasting longer than thirty minutes, pack perishable food such as meat, poultry, eggs, cheese, and salads with a freezer pack.

- Pack drinks in a separate cooler so the food cooler is not opened as frequently.

- Do not stow the cooler in the trunk of the car, which gets much hotter than the passenger compartment.

- Pack snacks from at least two food groups, and choose those that are low in added salt, sugar, and fat and are made from fewer processed ingredients.

- Avoid snacks that melt, crumble, stick, or dribble down chins.

- Pack individual snack/lunch bags for children or have them pick, prepare, and pack their own.

- Give kids several components to "build" a snack with, such as rice cakes, cheese, and fruit.

**Some snack suggestions:**

- For toddlers, stick with familiar finger foods, such as unsweetened organic cereal (e.g., Puffins); organic cheese sticks; rice cakes; or fresh fruit. Be sure not to pack choking hazards such as grapes, berries, raisins, nuts, and seeds, especially if you are driving and the child is in the backseat out of your reach.

- Elementary-age children may want to participate in packing their own snacks, especially if you have a special lunch box cooler for them. These include everything from the toddler list, plus carrot and celery sticks, applesauce cups, yogurt, popcorn, pretzels, trail mix, and fruit leathers.

- Children ages twelve and older can certainly participate in planning their snack meals and still avoid junk! They can pack energy bars, fruit/yogurt shakes, rice cakes, trail mix, and fresh fruit.

**If you are stuck at an airport:**

- Look for places that serve breakfast foods like eggs, oatmeal, and yogurt.

- Avoid high-sodium fast foods such as Chinese cuisine: When flying, your body retains water and the sodium effect will be more pronounced.

- Many newsstands sell energy bars. While not a substitute for good nutrition, they are better than chips and candy.

- Be sure your kids have plenty of water—avoid juices and energy drinks.

## They'll Do As You Do

If you want your kids to eat healthy, guess what? You've got to eat healthy, too. You can't expect them to give up chips and candy if you don't. And there's no way you can convince your children to try the spinach or broccoli if there are no vegetables on your plate. Make sure your portions are appropriate for you as well as your kids. If they see you overeating, they may try to copy your bad habits. Avoid weighing out portions, obsessively counting calories, or disparaging yourself for being overweight. Serve a variety of foods and let your kids know when you are stopping eating because you're feeling full.

Take heart from the fact that every family faces these same kinds of food issues, including the First Family. In a September 2009 issue of *Children's Health,* Michelle Obama stated that she had been trying to get her family to eliminate processed foods, cut back on sugary drinks, and eat more fresh fruits and vegetables. She also told interviewer Peter Moore that thinking about how her family ate had become part of her life because of her children. "We are their primary role models," she told Moore. "And if they see me exercising and thinking about what I'm eating, if they see their father, as busy as he is, getting to the gym and playing sports, when they grow up they'll understand that this is a natural part of being an adult."

## Questions to Ask Your Child's Doctor

- How can I get my child to vary her diet?

- Do you have any suggestions for my picky eater?

- Is my child anemic or in need of any extra vitamins or supplements?

- Are my child's teeth in good shape? When does he need to see a pediatric dentist?

# Chapter 12 Take-Home Points

- There is a lot we can do nutritionally to keep kids healthy. It's part of our job as parents, because how we feed our kids now and how we talk to them about what they eat can have a huge impact on their lifelong relationship with food.

- Talk to your kids about food and nutrition. Answer any questions they may have and let them know why some foods are healthier for them than others.

- Talk to your kids about commercials and advertising and the influence they have on our food choices.

- Try to have a family mealtime as often as possible, and make it a positive experience. It's not the time to lecture or scold your kids. It should be a calm, warm, and friendly time for the family to reconnect.

- Encourage your children to be involved in the planning and preparation of family meals. Talk to them about the various components that go into a balanced meal, and allow them to make choices in each category. Let them help shop for food and give them age-appropriate tasks for the meal.

- Avoid food battles. Establish routines and rules and stick to them. Allow your kids to have more of any food they're served, but don't make alternative meals if they won't eat what's on their plate.

- Don't negotiate with your children or use food as a reward.

- Remember that kids won't starve themselves. If they skip a meal one day, they'll eat again when they get hungry. Even picky eaters will eventually balance out their nutritional needs.

- Be a role model. Your children will follow your lead; they'll eat healthily if you do.

Even with all our good intentions, there are times when a child's eating issues may get out of control. Unfortunately, anorexia and bulimia have become all too familiar problems in our homes and schools, and obesity in children has become a national epidemic. The next chapter will talk about these issues, how to recognize them, and what you can do if they show up in your family.

# CHAPTER 13

# Disordered Eating and the Obesity Issue: How to Monitor Your Child's Eating Habits without Going Overboard

*Charlie is a nine-year-old boy who arrived in my office for the first time because his mother was worried he was "so fat and yet he never eats." With Charlie in the office, she reported that he eats only organic food, and he doesn't get candy or sweets. She says he exercises and still gets "fatter and fatter," and she is sure he has a thyroid problem. Charlie weighed 185 pounds on my office scale and measured 5 feet 2 inches. He seemed very anxious. Every time his mother began to talk, his face fell and he stared at the floor. I asked him some questions about his school and he barely answered.*

*Then I spoke to the mother alone: His breakfast? Homemade pancakes. His lunch? At school. His typical dinner? Fish or meat plus a vegetable and a starch. Number of servings? Three. Portion size? Huge. Juice? No, only smoothies. Exercise? Treadmill at home for fifteen minutes twice a week. TV? Only allowed two hours per night. Friends? Not many—he switched schools last year. Family activities? The movies. . . .*

*I did blood work to be sure that his thyroid was indeed normal and to check his B12, folate, magnesium, selenium, and other parameters of good nutrition. I put him on a multivitamin and an exercise program that was fun for him, not the torture of a treadmill for a nine-year-old boy. I recommended that he have at least one playdate a week, cut the TV time in half, and eat only one serving at dinner. Smoothies were to replace the pancakes in the morning, then only water the rest of the day. And, most important, I recommended that the entire family exercise together and eat more meals together to encourage happier and healthier mealtimes.*

*Charlie lost 25 pounds and is still working hard on his health. He took up karate and rock climbing. In addition, his father has lost 20 extra pounds and his mother 10.*

*—From Dr. Geary's files*

Parents today often find themselves between a rock and a hard place. It's difficult enough to manage their own weight problems without having to become the food police for their children's eating issues.

The last chapter was all about how to encourage your kids to develop healthy eating habits. This is advice we should all follow all the time. Sometimes, however, even the best of intentions don't pan out as planned. Because there are so many temptations and influences, both inside and outside the home, that kids have to deal with every day, it frequently seems an impossible task to keep your children nutritionally sound. After all, you're only in control over what your kids eat until they're about two years old. As they get older, they spend more and more time at day care, at playdates, at school, or with a nanny or caregiver. By the time they're four, five, or six years old, eating patterns are already established. And because we can't be with our kids 24/7, there is no easy fix.

In fact, a recent study showed that even children who had been taken to a doctor for help in losing weight didn't end up eating more fruit or vegetables or less fat, and they didn't lose significant amounts of weight. The researchers reported that brief, physician-led intervention produced no long-term improvement in body mass index, physical activity, or nutrition habits. Part of the reason for that is that kids don't really have a sense of their own mortality or long-term medical vulnerability. They have problems connecting the fact that eating broccoli and quinoa today can help them avoid heart disease when they're fifty. If adults, who do have a sense of their own mortality, have difficulty maintaining a nutritionally sound diet regimen, imagine how hard it is for kids.

Most of the time eating issues are complicated. It's not always as simple as serving your kids carrots in place of chips as snacks. Pediatricians don't always give helpful advice to parents of overweight kids, saying things like "Oh, just make sure your child eats more vegetables," or "Don't worry, he'll grow out of it." A lot of kids actually "grow into it," meaning that as they grow taller, they grow into their weight. But in many cases, emotional issues are involved as well as nutritional ones, and these need to be addressed.

That is not to say that nothing can be done to help your children eat healthy. Many of the techniques in the last chapter really do work. There are times, however, when a child's unhealthy eating habits go beyond what is acceptable deviation and turn into eating disorders. It is beyond the scope of this book to deal with eating disorders in great depth (there are entire books on the subject), but it's important for you to know when your kids are getting into nutritional trouble so that you can determine when it's a matter of helping your children make better choices and when it might be best to seek professional help.

## What Is an Eating Disorder?

Ask any number of health professionals for the meaning of *"eating disorder"* and you will get any number of different answers. Most of the definitions state that people with eating disorders have self-critical negative thoughts paired with unusual and unhealthy eating habits. There are only two eating disorders officially defined by the American Psychiatric Association to date: *anorexia nervosa* and *bulimia nervosa.*

Obviously, there are many other varieties of problems related to eating. We are referring to these problems as "disordered eating." While we will briefly outline both anorexia and bulimia later in the chapter (these disorders are affecting younger and younger children, and it's essential that parents become aware of the warning signs), we are concentrating here on the frighteningly rapid rise of childhood obesity in this country.

## THE OBESITY ISSUE

Obesity is the most prevalent nutritional disorder among children and adolescents in the United States. One out of every six kids is overweight, and 80 percent of those who are heavy as children will be heavy as adults.

How do you know what your child is supposed to weigh? After all, children have different body types and varying rates of growth and development. Put two kids of the same age, gender, and height next to each other and they can look like Mutt and Jeff even though they are both well within the normal weight range. Children also go through normal periods of growth spurts, especially during adolescence, when they put on weight rapidly as the amount of bone, muscle, and fat in their bodies changes. We've all seen the chubby twelve-year-old who lives on junk food and sporadically exercises yet naturally blossoms into a long and lean teenager. So just because your child has suddenly put on weight or doesn't conform to your standards of fitness doesn't mean that he or she is the one in six who is overweight.

Being overweight is usually defined by your child's doctor in terms of your child's growth curve: Does his height match his weight on the percentile curve? For example, suppose your child weighs 50 pounds at age eight, but is in the 95th percentile for height (which means that your child is taller than 95 percent of other children his age). This is very different than if your eight-year-old weighs 50 pounds and is in the 50th percentile for height.

There is another way health professionals can assess overweight and obesity; it's called the BMI or Body Mass Index. It's a formula (your weight divided by the square of your height) used to estimate how much body fat a person has based on his or her weight and height. For children, BMI is also calculated on a percentile system as in the chart below:

| Weight Status Category | Percentile Range |
| --- | --- |
| Underweight | Less than the 5th percentile |
| Healthy weight | 5th percentile to less than the 85th percentile |
| Overweight | 85th percentile to less than the 95th percentile |
| Obese | Equal to or greater than the 95th percentile |

Obviously, this is an imperfect system. BMI can be misleading in some situations. A muscular teen, for example, may have a high BMI without being overweight because extra muscle adds to body weight. There are many variables in children, whose actual percentages of body fat may vary by age, race, stage of development, height, and sexual maturity. These criteria are different from those used to interpret BMI for adults, which do not take into account age or sex. Age and sex are considered for children and teens for two reasons: The amount of body fat changes with age, and the amount of body fat differs between girls and boys.

### How to Measure Your Kids at Home

You can calculate your child's BMI yourself with the help of the Internet. The Centers for Disease Control and Prevention Web site (www.cdc.gov) provides a BMI calculator for children and teens. In order to use it, you need to have accurate measurements of your child's height and weight.

**To measure height accurately at home, follow these CDC guidelines:**

1. Remove the child's shoes, bulky clothing, and hair ornaments, and unbraid hair that interferes with the measurement.

2. Take the height measurement on flooring that is not carpeted and against a flat surface such as a wall with no molding.

3. Have the child stand with feet flat, together, and against the wall. Make sure legs are straight, arms are at sides, and shoulders are level.

4. Make sure the child is looking straight ahead and that the line of sight is parallel with the floor.

5. Take the measurement while the child stands with head, shoulders, buttocks, and heels touching the flat surface (wall).

Depending on the overall body shape of the child, all points may not touch the wall.

6. Place a flat headpiece, such as a book or a board, on the child's head to form a right angle with the wall. Lower the headpiece until it firmly touches the crown of the head.

7. Make sure your eyes are at the same level as the headpiece. If you're measuring a young child, you may have to kneel on the floor so that your eyes are at the level of the headpiece.

8. Lightly mark where the bottom of the headpiece meets the wall. Then, use a metal tape to measure from the base on the floor to the mark on the wall to get the height measurement.

9. Accurately record the height to the nearest ⅛ inch or 0.1 centimeter.

**To measure weight accurately at home to calculate BMI-for-age:**

1. Use a digital scale. Avoid using bathroom scales that are spring-loaded. Place the scale on firm flooring (such as tile or wood) rather than carpet.

2. Have the child or teen remove shoes and heavy clothing, such as sweaters.

3. Have the child or teen stand with both feet in the center of the scale.

4. Record the weight to the nearest decimal fraction (e.g., 55.5 pounds or 25.1 kilograms).

Once you have these accurate measurements, you can go to the CDC Web site at http://apps.nccd.cdc.gov/dnpabmi/ and follow the instructions for utilizing the BMI calculator for children and teens.

## *Scary Statistics*

According to national surveys, the number of children who are overweight in America has increased dramatically; in fact, the number has tripled since 1980. Some statistics say that more than 25 percent of children and adolescents are at risk or are already overweight, and more than 15 percent of children ages six to eighteen are considered obese. Perhaps the most frightening statistics are that approximately 80 percent of children who were overweight at ages ten to fifteen years were obese adults at the age of twenty-five, and that 25 percent of obese adults were overweight as children. Studies have also found that if children are overweight before the age of eight, they are likely to be more severely overweight as adults.

Using BMI calculations, the prevalence of overweight (BMI of 85th to 95th percentile) children and adolescents in the United States has increased by 50 to 60 percent in a single generation, and the prevalence of obesity has doubled.

## WHY IS YOUR CHILD OVERWEIGHT?

Good question. The simplest explanation is that he is taking in more calories than he uses to support normal growth and development, metabolism, and physical activity. But we all know that's not all there is to it. There are many factors, usually working in combination, that contribute to your child's weight:

### It's because of their genes.

- Does your daughter's body shape remind you of yourself, your mother, or your grandmother? Does your son's build mimic his father's? Heredity has a lot to do with it. Kids who come from different ethnicities, races, and nationalities often have different body shapes because they accumulate fat in different parts of their bodies. But it's important to note that our genetics have not changed for thousands of years. It's a very small factor in who is overweight and who isn't. The rate of rise in childhood obesity far surpasses the rate of change in genetics.

The genes we inherit from our ancestors are not the whole story—they mean you're predisposed, not predetermined. It's not your child's destiny to be overweight just because it runs in your family. Blaming weight on their genes makes kids think that there is nothing they can do to change their situation. In fact, there are many things we can do to change children's diet, bad habits, and activity levels to help them reach and keep a healthy weight.

**The genes we inherit from our ancestors are not the whole story—they mean you're predisposed, not predetermined. It's not your child's destiny to be overweight just because it runs in your family.**

### It's because of their food choices.

- Macaroni and cheese. Chicken fingers. Chips. Candy. Ice cream. We all know what the villains are. They're not hidden away in the cupboard; they're everywhere we turn. Kids naturally go for the sweetest, most calorie-laden foods they can get away with eating. There's no getting around the fact that fast foods and fat kids go together like burgers and fries, and there's no getting around the fact that these foods will make them fat.

### It's because of their beverage choices.

- One of the easiest ways to cut down on calories is to cut down on juice boxes. They're convenient and kids love them—but they're packed with calories and sugar. If you do give your kids juice, it should always be diluted. Kids don't need soda, diet or otherwise. And they don't need sports or energy drinks. All they really need to drink is water.

### It's because of what you teach them.

- You can't control every bit of what goes into your kids' mouths, especially as they get older. But who buys the food that's in your house? If you've got a pantry full of sweet, salty, and fatty foods, you can't blame your kids for eating them. Your unhealthy eating habits will be passed down to your children just as surely as your genes were.

### It's because of TV and video games.

- You don't burn many calories sitting in front of the television or the computer screen. It is estimated that children between the ages of eight and eighteen spend slightly more than three hours per day watching TV, videos, and DVDs—and many studies have found a direct correlation between time spent viewing television and the increased prevalence of obesity in children. Kids who watch more than four hours a day are more likely to be overweight compared with kids who watch two hours or less.

- It's not only the inactivity of watching TV that's a problem. A recent study found that kids ages seven to eleven ate 45 percent more while watching a half-hour cartoon interspersed with ads for food than those who watch the same cartoon with ads featuring nonfood items.

### It's because of socioeconomic factors.

- Poverty and obesity often go hand in hand. Let's face it, junk food costs a lot less than organic produce. Many schools that provide breakfast for underprivileged children feed them pastries and sugary sweets. Low-income families often do not have the time or the resources to make healthy eating and exercise a priority.

### It's because of the environment.

- There is a new culprit in the plethora of obesity villains, and it's called an obesogen (a chemical that disturbs a body's normal metabolic processes, causing it to tend toward obesity). In 2006, scientists at the Harvard School of Public Health reported that the prevalence of obesity in infants (yes, infants!) under six months had risen 73 percent since 1980. They began looking for causes, since it couldn't be blamed on junk food or too much TV.

One theory they came up with was exposure to environmental chemicals during development, including bisphenol A (BPA), a chemical used in making plastics and often used in making plastic baby bottles. Being exposed to BPA during development changes your body weight. Mice that were exposed to tiny amounts of BPA while in the womb gained more weight than mice that were not exposed. It turned out that each fat cell in the exposed mice actually had more fat in it. Obviously, not everyone who is overweight can use obesogens such as BPA, which is found in hundreds of consumer products, as an excuse. But it may help explain why some people can eat the same amount of food as their thinner friends and still put on the pounds.

## WHAT'S EATING OUR KIDS?

We can't talk about the obesity issue without discussing one of its major causes: emotional eating. We've all done it at one time or another. If we're feeling lonely, we turn to our friends Ben and Jerry. If we're overworked, we take a break and have some cake. Kids do it, too. They eat not only when they are hungry, but also to deal with feelings of anger, stress, boredom, happiness, depression, and any other feelings that come to mind. That's emotional eating: consuming unhealthy foods or unhealthy amounts of food in response to emotions instead of hunger.

Your child might be an emotional eater if he or she:

- Obsesses about food

- Eats impulsively

- Can't stop eating even when he's full

- Hides evidence of eating

- Eats at a faster-than-normal rate

- Expresses feelings of remorse after eating

- Avoids interaction at social events by eating

Emotional eating is a habit that children often learn at an early age—and usually learn from their parents. If your child has had a particularly bad day, you don't take her out for a plate of broccoli. You take her out for ice cream, or say, "Let's bake some cupcakes!" If you want your child to do something necessary but unpleasant, like getting a flu shot or vaccination, you promise him a stop at the donut shop on the way home. Happy occasions can be reasons for food-related celebrations as well. Good grades are often rewarded with fast food dinners or extra-special desserts. In this way, children learn that the way to deal with bad days and stressful events is to eat something unhealthy and/or to associate positive events with overindulgence.

**The best way to deal with emotional eating is to find a distraction.**

We're not saying that you should never take your children out for a treat. But perhaps you can more often reward them in other ways, such as a trip to the movies (sans the popcorn), a play, the zoo, or the park. Maybe you can buy them an inexpensive toy (you don't want to teach them they can buy their way out of emotional situations either). Or maybe you can just heap them with praise and give them a hug.

What can you do if you think your child is an emotional eater? Talk to your child's pediatrician or someone who specializes in eating issues immediately. Talk to your kids about when and why they eat. Help them make the connection between how they feel and why they eat. Ask them to fill out a food diary of what they are eating and when and what they were feeling at the time. Not every child will have the discipline to do this, but even if they do it for a few days, it may help them understand that they eat when they're angry or bored.

The best way to deal with emotional eating is to find a distraction. If your child is angry and wants to comfort herself with food, tell her to go to her room, shut the door, put on some loud music, and dance around. Play a game with your child or give her a puzzle to solve. Find something age-appropriate that will take her mind off eating. If it's possible to get her involved in some physical activity (riding a bike, raking the lawn, playing a sport), even better.

Occasional emotional eating is generally not a cause for concern, but when it becomes a habit it can also become a health concern that needs to be addressed.

## THE DANGERS OF CHILDHOOD OBESITY

If the statistics cited earlier weren't frightening enough, here's a statement that just may shock you: This generation of children who are overweight are not going to live as long as their parents.

Even with all the improvements in pharmaceuticals and medical care that have been developed over the last several decades, this is the first time scientists are warning that this generation is in danger of dying at younger ages than their parents will. This is because overweight and obese children and teens can develop serious health problems starting in childhood and carrying over into their adult years. Here are just some of the health issues these kids may experience:

> **This generation of children who are overweight are not going to live as long as their parents.**

### *Metabolic Syndrome*

Metabolic syndrome is a cluster of conditions that occur together. You (or your child) may be diagnosed with metabolic syndrome if you have at least three of the following conditions:

- High blood pressure

- Insulin resistance

- Abdominal obesity

- High blood sugar

- Low HDL (good) cholesterol

- High triglycerides (fats in the blood)

- Inflammatory reactions in the blood

Abdominal obesity and insulin resistance are the most dominant risk factors for metabolic syndrome. Insulin resistance is a condition where the body can't use insulin efficiently; therefore, metabolic syndrome is also sometimes called the insulin resistance syndrome. People with metabolic syndrome are at increased risk of coronary heart disease, stroke, peripheral vascular disease, and type 2 diabetes. Metabolic syndrome is on the rise in the United States. Approximately fifty million Americans may have it, and it is increasingly being diagnosed in children as the incidence of obesity rises.

### Diabetes

Diabetes, also known as diabetes mellitus, is a disease in which your body does not use or produce insulin properly. Insulin is an important hormone necessary for the absorption of blood sugar, also known as glucose. If there is too much glucose in your blood, it can lead to serious health complications. There are two types of diabetes. Type 1 diabetes has nothing to do with being overweight or obese. It occurs suddenly when your immune system attacks and destroys the insulin-producing cells in the pancreas. Type 2 diabetes develops over time and occurs when your cells become resistant to insulin. This type of diabetes used to be called "adult-onset" diabetes; however, because more and more children and adolescents are being diagnosed with this form of diabetes, that designation is no longer in use. Even twenty years ago, most doctors never saw children who had type 2 diabetes. While studies suggest that type 2 diabetes in children and adolescents is still relatively rare, it is being diagnosed more frequently, particularly in Native American, African American, and Hispanic and Latino American populations.

If not treated, diabetes can cause severe complications down the line, including heart disease and stroke, kidney disease, blindness and other eye problems, gum disease, foot problems, and even depression. One of the problems with type 2 diabetes in both children and adults is that some people with the disease never even know they have it because they experience no signs or symptoms. However, some do experience symptoms such as:

- Increased thirst and frequent urination

- Increased hunger

- Weight loss (despite eating more than usual to relieve hunger, your child may lose weight)

- Fatigue

- Blurred vision

- Slow-healing sores or frequent infections

- Areas of darkened skin, usually in the armpits and neck (This condition, called *acanthosis nigricans*, may be a sign of insulin resistance.)

The only way to know for sure if your child has diabetes is to have her tested by a physician. If your child's BMI is in the 85th percentile or higher, it's a good idea to have her tested. The good news about type 2 diabetes is that it can be well controlled and sometimes even reversed by losing weight, exercising, and following a healthy eating plan.

### Cardiovascular Disease

A recent study conducted by researchers at the Nemours Children's Clinic in Jacksonville, Florida, and the Mayo Clinic in Rochester, Minnesota, found that the unhealthy consequences of excess body fat can start very early. The study included 115 obese children with a BMI above the 95th percentile, as well as 87 lean children as controls. The participants were children between the ages of seven and eighteen who had normal fasting blood sugar levels (meaning they did not have diabetes) and did not have metabolic syndrome. The researchers were looking for known markers for predicting the development of cardiovascular disease. They found that the obese children, even those as young as seven, had a ten times higher incidence of these markers than the lean children did.

### *Heightened Estrogen Levels*

The enzyme that converts testosterone into estrogen (aromatase) resides primarily in the fat cells. The more fat you carry, the more estrogen you will produce, which may increase the risk of breast cancer later on in life.

### *Nonalcoholic Fatty Liver Disease (NAFLD)*

Nonalcoholic fatty liver disease is now believed to be due to insulin resistance, which is closely associated with obesity. In fact, the BMI correlates with the degree of liver damage; that is, the greater the BMI the greater the liver damage. NAFLD can lead to a wide spectrum of liver diseases ranging from fatty liver syndrome to hepatitis and cirrhosis.

### *Social and Emotional Problems*

Children who are overweight or obese often suffer from social and emotional fallout. They are frequently teased and bullied by other children, which causes them to have low self-esteem. This also puts them at high risk for depression and school-related anxiety. The result is that they either become socially withdrawn and have trouble making friends, or they act out in school and disrupt the classroom. Either way, they end up with learning problems.

### Overweight children are also at risk of developing:

- High blood pressure

- Asthma and other respiratory problems

- Sleep disorders

- Early puberty or menarche

- Skin infections

- Eating disorders

According to the American Council for Fitness and Nutrition, "being overweight at a young age appears to be far more destructive to well-being than adding excess pounds in later life." No wonder parents are so concerned about their overweight children! All of this information can be disheartening and discouraging. Fortunately, there are steps you can take to help prevent and treat obesity. Truthfully, it won't always be easy. But by following the suggestions in the next section and not expecting overnight results, you can help your child back on the road to a healthier life.

## What Can Be Done for an Overweight Child?

Helping someone else to lose weight is always a tricky task, no matter what the person's age. Everyone is sensitive about their weight. Children are super sensitive, and anything you say can be taken as an insult and an indication that you don't love them as you should. It doesn't matter whether these things are true or not, it just matters that this is the way your child feels.

> For most children weight should be maintained as they grow up in height, as opposed to using calorie restriction to lose significant weight.

The best way to help your child lose weight is the tried-and-true method: You have to make changes in your child's diet and level of physical activity. Before you make any changes, however, you should take your child to the doctor. Have the doctor measure your child's BMI and note if there has been a marked increase in the last year. There may be tests that your doctor recommends to rule out any medical problems that may be causing weight gain.

Do not make your child "diet." Putting a child on a diet is usually not considered safe practice. Of course, this is more difficult if they have already gone through puberty. But for most children, weight should be maintained as they grow up in height, as opposed to using calorie restriction to lose significant weight. If your child is eight years old and already 100 pounds, you don't want him to lose any weight. You want him to stay 100 pounds as he becomes nine and ten and eleven and twelve and gets taller every year. This requires great patience on the part of parents, but in the end will be the safest way for your child to learn to manage food and weight. If it has been established that your child is overweight, there are many steps you can take instead of putting your child on a strict diet:

- **Take charge of mealtime.** You're the parent. For the most part, you're the one who buys and cooks the food and decides what is available for snacks and treats. Limit the amount of juices and sweetened drinks in the house. Make sure there are plenty of fruits and vegetables as well as quality proteins. Keep track of the amount of wheat or wheat products as well as dairy and dairy products your child is consuming, and try to limit those as well, especially in one twenty-four-hour period. Provide children with a variety of foods to ensure they get all the nutrients they need for proper growth and development, and keep portion sizes in check to help children maintain their sense of self-regulation and to know when they are hungry and when they are full. Follow the recommendations from Part II of this book and your child will have balanced, nutritious meals every time.

- **Get your child moving.** Active children are more likely to become fit adults. Physical activity not only burns calories, it also helps build strong bones and muscle. It helps kids sleep at night and focus during the day. Exercise has also been shown to help lower triglycerides and blood pressure (we will go into the importance of exercise in more depth in Chapter 14).

- **Limit TV and video time.** For kids ages two and up the American Academy of Pediatrics (AAP) recommends limiting time spent in front of a screen to no more than two hours per day. The AAP also discourages any screen time for children younger than two years.

- **Don't let your kids skip breakfast.** When you skip breakfast (or any other meal), you slow your resting metabolic rate—the number of calories your body burns at rest. Metabolism is the process whereby the body converts food into energy, uses it for repairs, or stores it as fat for future use. In simple terms, a faster metabolism burns calories more efficiently and stores less fat. A slower metabolism burns calories less efficiently and therefore causes more calories to be stored as fat. You want to speed up your metabolism at the start of the day, which ideally means including a high-quality protein as part of the meal.

- **Know what they get to eat in school.** Unfortunately, meals offered by schools are not as healthy as they should be. If you can, go over the school menu with your children and help them make decisions about the choices they are going to make for lunch. They may follow them, or they may not, but at least you will have gotten them talking about healthy meals. Or pack them a healthy lunch that includes a quality protein, a veggie or two, and fruit for dessert.

### Which Is Healthier, A4 or G12?

A decade ago, vending machines in schools were rare indeed. But principals and parents slowly began to recognize them as a source of revenue to pay for things like computer labs, sports programs, and after-school activities. Many of these machines, however, offer a variety of sugary and/or salt-laden snacks and drinks. You can do your part by complaining to the school or school board about these unhealthy offerings. In 2009, the New York City Education Department mandated that schools promote healthier choices for students. Drinks sold in vending machines in elementary and middle schools must have fewer than 10 calories per 8 ounces. In high school, drinks must have fewer than 25 calories per 8 ounces. No artificially sweetened drinks or sodas are allowed. Drinks have to be caffeine-free or non-carbonated; for example, water, seltzer, or sugar-free tea. Snacks were also subject to limits on calories and fat and sugar content. If you don't like what's in your schools, get together with other parents to push for changes and healthier choices. This may not be the ultimate solution to the obesity epidemic, but it is a start.

- **Lead by example.** Your kid will do what you do. You can't recommend that your kid try new foods if you turn up your nose at turnips. You can't expect her to go out and play if you never get out of your computer chair. If you stay active and eat a balanced diet, your child is more likely to follow your lead.

- **Concentrate on positive feedback.** Remind your child that food should not ruin his day or dominate his life—it's just a piece of food. And keep in mind that if you're constantly focused on your child's weight, it may just backfire and cause your child to eat more or to develop an eating disorder. Take the weight issue seriously, but lighten up.

- **Love your children unconditionally.** Emphasize the fact that you love them no matter what they weigh and that you want them to be healthy and happy as they grow and mature.

### ANOREXIA AND BULIMIA

We live in a strange country where there is an epidemic of obesity at the same time that our culture reveres thinness, especially for young women. Teens, tweens, and young adults in Hollywood are outed every time they gain a few pounds. Paparazzi constantly focus on their flaws. Magazines airbrush the flaws away so that young readers believe these starlets are perfect and that they themselves will never measure up to society's standards. Some children have a difficult time facing the dramatic physical changes and societal pressures they encounter as they hit puberty. They sometimes sadly resort to the two eating disorders officially defined by the American Psychiatric Association to date: *anorexia nervosa* and *bulimia nervosa*.

Boys are affected, too, although eating disorders are more common among girls. Both boys and girls with eating disorders have a distorted image of how they actually look. They may be quite thin, and yet see themselves as overweight. If they engage in certain sports and activities like gymnastics, ballet, cheerleading, wrestling, or ice skating, they may feel great pressure to reach or maintain a certain weight.

One of the most disturbing aspects of these eating disorders is that they are showing up in younger and younger children. The Centers for Disease Control and the National Association of Eating Disorders report that 42 percent of first- to third-grade girls want to be thinner, 82 percent of ten-year-olds are afraid of being fat, more than 50 percent of today's teenage girls are on diets and use unhealthy means to control their weight, and most kids with eating disorders began when they were between the ages of eight and thirteen.

**Anorexia and bulimia are not fads or stages that will go away on their own. They are serious disorders, and require professional help.**

Anorexia and bulimia are not fads or stages that will go away on their own. They are serious disorders, and require professional help.

### *Anorexia*

People with anorexia, a life-threatening disorder, literally try to starve themselves. They are obsessed with food, even though they don't eat very much at all. It is a way of dealing with the conflicts, pressures, and stresses of their lives. Anorexia may be used as a way to express control when the rest of one's life seems out of control.

There are warning signs that your child may be suffering from anorexia. A person who is suffering from anorexia might:

- Become very thin, frail, or emaciated and may end up losing 15 percent or more of her ideal body weight

- Go on a strict diet even though he is not overweight

- Have a distorted body image, constantly complaining about how fat she is even when she is thin or underweight

- Be obsessed with food, calories, nutrition, or cooking

- Deny that he is hungry

- Exercise obsessively

- Weigh himself repeatedly

- Exhibit loss of hair or thinning hair

- Feel cold all the time even in warm temperatures

- Stop menstruating

- Be depressed, lethargic, or withdraw from social activities, especially those that involve food

Anorexia can cause heart and kidney problems; a drop in blood pressure, pulse, and breathing rate; growth of soft hair all over the skin; lightheadedness and an inability to concentrate; anemia; swollen joints; and brittle bones. It can lead to malnutrition and even death.

### Bulimia

Bulimia is also a life-threatening disorder. Characterized by a pattern of binge eating and purging (which can involve extreme exercising, vomiting, or use of laxatives), it is sometimes more difficult to spot because bulimics go through weight fluctuations, but do not usually become thin or emaciated like anorexics. Bulimics may even be overweight. Women with bulimia often feel out of control in other areas of their lives besides food. They may spend money excessively, abuse drugs or alcohol, or engage in chaotic relationships.

There are warning signs that your child may be suffering from bulimia. A person who is suffering from bulimia might:

- Engage in binge eating and not be able to stop

- Use the bathroom frequently after meals

- Experience frequent fluctuations in weight

- React to emotional stress by overeating

- Regularly buy laxatives, diuretics, or enemas

- Have menstrual irregularities

- Have swollen glands

- Spend an excessive amount of time running, going to the gym, or working out

- Be obsessively concerned about weight

- Feel guilty or ashamed about eating

- Be depressed or withdraw from social activities, especially those that involve food

Bulimia can cause constant stomach pain, dental and esophageal problems, kidney damage, heartburn, chemical imbalance (including loss of potassium, which can contribute to heart problems), and an overall loss of energy and vitality. It can even prove fatal.

## WHAT CAN YOU DO?

The most important steps you can take if you suspect that your child has an eating disorder are to talk to your child and to seek professional help. Children with eating disorders often get very defensive and angry if confronted about them. They might not even be able to admit they have a problem. Don't accuse them of doing something wrong: "You're not eating enough" or tell them they look terrible: "You're getting so thin I can hardly look at you." Instead, tell them that you're concerned that they're losing weight too quickly or that you can see how difficult it must be to count every calorie. Let them know that going to the doctor will help put your mind at ease.

Monitor your child's Internet use. Unfortunately, there are Web sites devoted to such disturbing topics as how to be a better anorexic. If you do find your child has visited such a site, discuss it calmly and ask what they saw and felt when looking at such information.

Examine your own attitudes about beauty and weight. Do you tell your child that he or she is getting fat? Do you criticize her weight, shape, or size? Or your own? Do you make fun of other people's weight, shape, or size?

As always, set an example for your kids. Don't panic if they don't want to eat certain foods or suddenly decide to become vegetarian. Give them love and support and let them know you'll do whatever you can to help them feel better about themselves.

# Questions to Ask Your Child's Doctor

- Is my child growing along a consistent growth curve for weight and height?

- What is my child's weight gain or loss in the last six months and is it normal?

- Is my child developing normally as he or she approaches or enters puberty?

- Is my teenage daughter's menses on schedule and is it normal for her age?

- At what point would you worry about my child's weight? At what point is it a medical risk?

- Should my child have his or her thyroid checked to be sure it is normal?

- Should my child be tested for diabetes?

- Who should help my child with his or her potential eating disorder or emotional eating?

- Should I share my concerns with my child's school? With her grandparents or other caretakers?

# Chapter 13 Take-Home Points

- Studies suggest that, for the first time in recent history, this generation of children who are overweight are not going to live as long as their parents.

- Obesity is the most prevalent nutritional disorder among children and adolescents in the United States. One out of every six kids is overweight, and 80 percent of those who are heavy as children will be heavy as adults.

- Being overweight is defined by your child's doctor in terms of your child's growth curve: Does his height match his weight on the percentile curve? The other way health professionals can assess overweight and obesity is by measuring Body Mass Index. It's a formula (your weight divided by the square of your height) used to estimate how much body fat a person has based on his or her weight and height.

- There are many factors, usually working in combination, that contribute to your child's weight, including the genes they have inherited from you and your mate; the food choices they make; the beverage choices they make (one of the easiest ways to cut down on calories is to cut down on juice boxes); what you teach them (your unhealthy eating habits will be passed down to your children just as surely as your genes were); how much time they spend in front of computer and TV screens; socioeconomic factors (poverty and obesity often go hand in hand); and the environment (exposure to environmental chemicals during fetal development).

- One of the major causes of obesity is emotional eating, which is eating to fill an emotional void or to avoid feeling the emotion at all (e.g., eating when angry, stressed, bored, happy, depressed, and any other feeling that comes to mind). The best way to deal with your child's emotional eating is to find a distraction. Find something age-appropriate that will take her mind off eating.

- What can be done for your overweight child? Take charge of mealtime. Get your child moving. Limit TV and video time. Don't let your kids skip breakfast. Know what they eat in school. Lead by example. Concentrate on positive feedback and love your children unconditionally.

- Educate yourself about eating disorders and recognize that they are showing up in younger and younger children. Familiarize yourself with the warning signs of anorexia and bulimia and know that the most important steps you can take if you suspect that your child has an eating disorder are to talk to your child and to seek professional help.

The thrust of this book has been all about nutrition. But as we all know, food isn't the only factor that goes into forming a healthy child. The next chapter takes a brief look at sleep, stress, and exercise, all of which are important aspects of a child's well-being.

# CHAPTER 14

# Adjuncts to Nutritional Wellness: Stress Relief, Sleep, and Exercise

You may wonder if all that you have read thus far is ever really going to be possible to incorporate into your family's lifestyle. It takes a long time to teach a child new habits, even longer for adults. But little by little, if you are willing to make small, simple changes to your child's nutrition (and maybe your own as well), you will find that your child is calmer, more grounded, less prone to illness, and is a happier and better performing student at school.

But what do you do if your child shows signs of exhaustion, irritability, stomachaches, and other symptoms we've talked about, but her food is fine? Although the main emphasis of this book is on nutrition, there are other areas of wellness that need to be addressed in order to ensure your child's overall health, including stress relief, sleep, and exercise. This chapter will be a roundup of the most important information and advice on these subjects.

What does wellness really mean for a child? Wellness is a state of being that focuses on balance and health rather than disease and treatment. The emphasis is on promoting the mind, body, and spirit in a way that is peaceful, easy, and consistent. In essence, it means practicing all the things that keep one well; it involves not just maintaining good nutrition, but also exercise, stress-control, sleep management, and good personal and familial social relationships. It is about your child's temperament (his natural manner of thinking, behaving, and reacting to life's situations) coming into balance with his constitution, an old-fashioned word that refers to your child's physical characteristics of health and strength.

## STRESS: IT'S NOT JUST FOR GROWN-UPS ANYMORE

It seems more and more impossible in our society to relax. People spend increasing amounts of money on "stress management," both at home and at work. Companies that specialize in providing programs and products for stress relief are hugely successful because everyone is so stressed out. And sadly, in both our practices, we see children and young adults already in the cycle of anxiety, stress, and depression that stems from the feeling of being overwhelmed.

You probably know that feeling all too well: tired, cranky, overwhelmed by your job, your bills, by a to-do list that never seems to get done, and even by your parenting responsibilities. Much as you try not to let it all show, your children feel the tension. And they learn the same responses: They become irritable, weepy, moody, and uncooperative. Finally, they do the one thing that you can't do—and that adds more stress to your day—they just lie down on the floor, kick, scream, and have a tantrum.

Although we think of stress as an emotion, it has direct physical consequences on your child's body. It can cause a hypervigilant flight reaction: Her heart races, her palms sweat, her breathing becomes rapid, and she becomes cranky, impatient, and, underneath it all, vulnerable to injury and illness. Dozens of studies over the years have shown the direct impact of stress on the immune system and how both children and adults under stress are much more prone to both acute and chronic illnesses.

It's hard to imagine that children feel stressed before they even start facing the massive amount of homework thrown at them in middle school. But studies have shown that even preschoolers feel stress. In fact, researchers at Washington University recently found that toddlers who feel overwhelmed or anxious can become depressed and carry that depression into middle school. We imagine that our young ones are oblivious to the pressures of life or that we can protect them from stress, but in fact they are often mirrors of the stress around them, from parents, caregivers, and teachers, to even "road ragers" yelling at each other out of car windows.

### *Where Does All That Stress Come From?*

While experts don't necessarily agree whether or not children today are more stressed than previous generations, we do know that younger and younger children are being pushed to be little adults, especially where getting good grades and getting into good schools is concerned. Our kids are certainly exposed to more violence than ever before, tend to spend more time away from their parents than any previous generation, and are exposed to and participate in more sexual activity at earlier ages than ever before.

If you think your child is stressed and you're trying to figure out why, here's a questionnaire that might help:

Has the family relocated recently? Yes ❏   No ❏

Has a parent lost his or her job? Yes ❏   No ❏

Are you going through a divorce or separation? Yes ❏   No ❏

Is there a lot of arguing in the house, between adults or among siblings? Yes ❏   No ❏

Is anyone in the family sick or injured? Yes ❏   No ❏

Have there been any difficulties in the family with alcohol or drug abuse? Yes ❏   No ❏

Has there been a recent death of a friend or member of the family? Yes ❏   No ❏

Has a pet passed away recently? Yes ❏   No ❏

Is the child being teased at school for any reason? Yes ❏   No ❏

Does your child have more homework than he or she can comfortably handle? Yes ❏   No ❏

Remember, having a stressed child is not something to be ashamed of. It often means that your child is more mature than you think and is processing information you thought you had shielded from him. Just like you hide your tears and worries from your child, he may be trying to hide his stress from you.

### *Warning Signs*

How can you tell if your child is having trouble with stress? Some of the signs are very obvious; others, not so much. Your child may be under stress if he or she:

- Becomes excessively whiny, clingy, and/or fearful

- Develops insomnia

- Becomes withdrawn and quiet and rarely laughs

- Displays a sudden onset of stuttering

- Is easily upset by any change in schedule or routine

- Loses his or her appetite or alternatively begins to hoard food

- Develops recurring headaches

- Has a chronic cough or stomach pains that usually go away on weekends

Sometimes a stressed-out child will regress by wetting the bed or sucking her thumb, hitting his friends, or refusing to go to school. If your child starts falling down and getting hurt more frequently, it may be because he is anxious and distracted. And if your child starts getting more ear infections, colds, and sore throats, it may be that stress is depressing her immune system. Children are especially vulnerable during their toddler and early childhood years because the hormones released when the body is under stress (e.g., cortisol) can affect brain development and delay growth.

**If your child starts falling down and getting hurt more frequently, it may be because he is anxious and distracted. And if your child starts getting more ear infections, colds, and sore throats, it may be that stress is depressing her immune system.**

Children, depending on their ages, don't necessarily recognize that they are stressed out; even older children and teens may have trouble verbalizing what's bothering them. That's why they're more likely to act out in school or at home. They may get into fights with their friends. Sometimes what seems like a behavioral problem is really a sign that your child needs help with stress management.

### De-Stressing Your Stressed-Out Kids

So what happens when your normally happy-go-lucky kid suddenly turns into a wrecking ball with a whiny streak? Is there anything you can do about it besides waiting for it to pass?

The first thing you should do is take a look in the mirror and ask yourself some tough questions. What is the general mood in your house? Are you and/or your significant other constantly stressed out? **Children often copy what they see going on around them and pick up the unhealthy vibrations they feel from their parents and caregivers. It may be that you need to learn to deal with your stress before you can help your children learn to deal with theirs.**

The best way to deal with your child's stress is to talk to him. You may be able to do this at family mealtime when everyone is sitting around the table. Not only will you encourage better nutrition and eating habits (see Chapter 12), but it also gives you an opportunity to casually and nonintrusively ask about the things on your child's mind. Remember, too, that misinformation is always worse than no information—and kids tend to be filled with misinformation from the playground.

### What Could Possibly Be Worrying Her?

*Maya was an eleven-year-old preteen whom I met while teaching her class the required sixth grade sexual education seminars. At the end of each session I asked the children to write anonymous questions on a piece of paper and put them in a box so I could read them and answer them without embarrassing anyone. One day, the following question came up: "I was told that if I got my period before age eleven I would get breast cancer. Is this true?"*

*I read this question out loud and answered, "Absolutely not. Girls get their periods anywhere from age nine to sixteen, which is considered the normal range. Certain ethnic groups get their periods earlier than others but it is not a risk factor for breast cancer."*

*Maya burst into tears in the middle of the classroom and her face shone with relief. She had been worrying about this for many months but had been afraid to ask her mother or another adult about it. Misinformation at this age is very powerful and can lead to significant amounts of distress.*

*—From Dr. Geary's files*

Be aware, though, that sometimes a stressed-out child may be more inclined to talk to you one-on-one than in front of his or her siblings. If you sense your child is uneasy, don't push him to share. Let him play a video game, relax in his room, maybe even help you cook dinner. Wait until he has had some downtime before broaching the subject of "what's on your mind" or "you seem like you had a hard day."

Coming home should be a relief for your child, a place where she feels safe both physically and emotionally. It should be a place where each one of you reiterates positive aspects about the other members of the family. Make simple statements like "I missed you today." "I love you so much." "I'm proud of you for how hard you're working." This should be a daily mantra for your kids to hear from you. Then you can say, "Tell me about your day." Be sure you take the time to actually listen to what they have to say.

If you are worried that your child may be stressed, consider these tips:

- **Explain what feeling "stressed" means.** Tell him that there are times in life when certain pressures build up, and that it is normal to worry. Try to help him identify what it is that is worrying him and ask him if he needs help in solving the problem.

- **Teach your child an emotional vocabulary.** When your child seems worried or nervous, you might say, "You seem anxious." Or when she is mad you can say, "You seem very upset." The particular words don't matter as long as you and all your child's caretakers are consistent. This will help your child to identify the feelings she has with words and later make her feel more in control and better able to express herself.

- **Help her to feel more in control of her world.** Review her day's agenda; let her know if there are big events coming up; include her in the planning for the week with visual clues like stickers and a big calendar she can work on with you.

- **Set aside special private time.** Spend some time alone with your child so he knows you are 100 percent focused on him and can really listen to his problems. This is particularly important if there is more than one child in the house—each sibling should feel that there are times when he or she gets your full attention.

- **Do not always try to solve the problem.** Just listen. This is essential to your child feeling like you have the time to listen without needing to "fix it" and thereby dismissing his anxiety. As a parent, it is natural to want to make things better for your children, but sometimes just listening and empathizing is really what they need.

- **Follow a routine as best you can.** Whether it's a bath time game or the ritual of reading the same book or listening to a particular piece of music or song, a child can find it very calming to know what to expect.

- **Teach simple stress relievers.** Explain that whenever she starts to feel stressed or anxious, she can stop what she's doing, sit still for a minute, and concentrate on her breathing.

- **Don't minimize their concerns.** No matter how small or trivial a thing your child is worried about, don't tell her she's being ridiculous or silly or being a baby. Let her know you understand how she's feeling and try and get her to tell you what it is about the situation that worries her. Then you can usually come up with a solution together.

The more worried and anxious you are, the more your kids will reflect your attitude, and before you know it, a vicious cycle is born. If simple techniques like the ones above are not working and stress is causing your child ongoing problems such as emotional distress, behavioral problems, or frequent illness, it's a good idea to seek help from a medical professional.

## SLEEP: BEDTIME BATTLES AND BOUNDARIES

Studies have shown that children, from elementary school to high school, get about an hour less sleep each night than they did thirty years ago, a deficiency that has the power to set their cognitive abilities back years. Because children's brains are continuously developing, and because much of that development happens when they are asleep, this lost hour appears to have an exponential impact on children that it doesn't have on adults (although adults are suffering from lack of sleep as well). It has even been theorized that many of the characteristics we normally associate with adolescence—moodiness, depression, and eating issues—are actually symptoms of chronic sleep deprivation. Sleep deprivation can lead to attention and behavioral issues in children, and it can affect their memories and their emotional well-being. Not to mention that children who sleep less are generally fatter than children who sleep more.

### Snooze and Lose

You might think that sleeping more would lead to weight gain because you spend all that time being inactive. But studies have shown otherwise, especially for children. Apparently, when you lose sleep your body increases the production of the hormone gherlin, which signals hunger. At the same time, it decreases the production of the hormone leptin, which suppresses appetite.

Cortisol, the stress hormone, rises with lack of sleep, and cortisol stimulates your body to make fat. Lastly, human growth hormone (HGH), so important for a child's development, which is secreted during sleep, is also essential for the breakdown of fat. It can't do its job properly if you're not getting enough sleep. So if your child is sleep deprived, all those hormones get out of whack and add to the risks of childhood obesity.

### How Much Sleep Do Children Need?

Sleep is probably one of the most discussed—and most argued about—aspects of child rearing. Expectant parents anticipate the worst in terms of their newborns' sleep patterns and their own sleep deprivation. Parents of children from toddlers to teens have related horror stories of children's bedtime battles that sometimes last for years. And parents everywhere worry that their kids are just not getting enough shuteye.

How much sleep is the right amount? That depends on the child's age, and on the child herself. Two children of the same age who get the same number of sleep hours may react quite differently, one needing more sleep than the other. But there are certain predictable ranges you can use to guide you in judging how much sleep your child probably needs:

- **From newborn to six months:** Before three months of age, babies are on their own particular schedules. Their internal clocks are not yet developed. They sleep about sixteen or seventeen hours a day, and can sleep for anywhere from one to five hours at a time. By the time they are three months old, they sleep about five hours during the day and ten hours at night with one or two interruptions, which means they usually sleep at least six or eight hours in a row, allowing parents to finally get some sleep themselves.

- **From six to twelve months:** At six months, babies average about eleven hours of sleep at night, and may nap for about three hours during the day. By this time, if they wake up during the night they should be able to go back to sleep on their own.

- **From one to three years:** Children of this age range may start to develop separation anxiety and put up a fight at bedtime. They need between ten and fourteen hours of sleep. Some toddlers may need daytime naps, but for others a short quiet time may be all that is needed.

---

### Perchance to Dream

Although scientists now believe that babies dream from the day they're born (and maybe even in the womb!), dreams can be pretty scary for toddlers who can't always tell the difference between what is real and what they have dreamt. It's important to monitor what movies or TV shows they watch before they go to bed, because animated monsters or villains will often show up in their dreams. If your child wakes up crying or screaming from a bad dream, let him talk about it if he wants to, and reassure him it was only in his imagination. Stay with him until he calms down, then encourage him to go back to sleep.

---

- **From four to six years:** These children need between ten and twelve hours of sleep per night. By the age of four, most children no longer need naps.

- **From six to nine years:** The average sleep requirement for this age range is about ten hours of sleep per night. This is also a time when many kids need some quiet private time with a parent, without brothers or sisters around. It may be that they have something they want to confide, or they just need a little one-on-one attention.

- **From ten to twelve years:** These children need between nine and eleven hours of sleep a night, but this can vary greatly from child to child. If your preteen child is particularly irritable or hyperactive, it just might be due to sleep deprivation.

- **Teenagers:** Because their bodies are going through so many changes, teens usually need between nine and nine-and-a-half hours a night. They don't usually get it, however. They stay up later at night and get up earlier. Although they often try to make up for lost sleep time on the weekends, this is not an adequate replacement for a regular sleep routine.

### How to Help Your Kids Get the Sleep They Need

There's nothing like that feeling you get when the day's pressures are over, the kids have bathed and brushed their teeth, and they are finally—finally—asleep in their very own beds. It's a chance to wind down, relax, and have that little bit of "me time" you've been craving all day. But sometimes those seemingly inevitable bedtime battles are so exhausting you have no energy left to do anything but watch a tiny bit of TV and fall into bed yourself. There are ways to make it easier for your child to get to sleep (and easier for you to get some downtime as well). Here are a few suggestions:

**Don't wait until your baby is asleep to put her to bed.**
- Put her in her crib when she's drowsy but still awake. This will help her learn to go back to sleep by herself if she wakes up in the night.

**If your infant wakes up crying, take a few minutes before you respond.**
- If the crying continues, go into the room to check on him, but don't turn on the light, don't pick him up or play with him. If he goes on crying, think about whether he might be hungry, need a diaper change, or if he might not be feeling well. If you do need to change a diaper or give him a bottle, do it as quickly and quietly as possible. Talk to the baby as little as possible; a

few words of comfort are all that are necessary. The less stimulation he gets, the easier it will be for him to go back to sleep.

**If your toddler cries or calls out to you during the night, wait several minutes before you respond.**
- If you do need to go into the room, don't turn on the light and don't stay in the room. Reassure your child that you're there but that it's time to go to sleep. If he calls out again, wait a longer time before responding and try speaking to him softly without entering the room again.

**Don't give your baby or toddler a bottle to help her fall asleep.**
- Children who fall asleep with a bottle of milk, juice, or any sweetened liquid in the mouth can suffer from a serious dental problem called "baby bottle tooth decay," because the fluids tend to pool in the child's mouth and can cause cavities in their front teeth.

**Keep your child's bedroom cool.**
- Everybody follows the circadian rhythm, which helps regulate sleep cycles. It is sensitive to light—we sleep when it's dark and wake when it's light. Turns out, it's temperature sensitive as well. If a room is too warm, sleep patterns change. We get less deep REM sleep, the state in the normal sleep cycle during which dreams occur and the body undergoes marked changes including rapid eye movement, loss of reflexes, and increased pulse rate and brain activity.

**Establish a bedtime routine.**
- This is probably the most valuable sleep aid you can provide. Make bedtime the same time every night. As we said earlier in the stress section, children like predictability and they want to know what to expect. Set up a quiet (the operative word here being *quiet*—no games or roughhousing before bed) routine

that you follow every night, such as reading a story or listening to soft music. A recent study in the *Journal of Developmental & Behavioral Pediatrics* found that those children who do not have consistent bedtime routines often develop later difficulties with sleep quality, duration, and timing, factors known to be associated with behavioral, cognitive, and health problems.

- It's not just children who benefit from bedtime routines. Another study published in the journal *Sleep* compared two groups of mothers and children. One group had been assigned a specific bedtime routine; the other was to follow their child's usual bedtime habits. The results? The bedtime routine resulted in significant reductions in problematic sleep behaviors for infants and toddlers, including how long it took them to fall asleep and the number of times they woke up in the night. Equally as important, the mothers in the routine group reported that their moods significantly improved. These results suggest that instituting a consistent nightly bedtime routine is beneficial in improving multiple aspects of infant and toddler sleep, and is a good thing for mom as well.

## THE IMPORTANCE OF EXERCISE

In 2009, children in America ages two to five watched more than thirty-two hours of television each week. Kids ages six to eleven watched a bit less—more than twenty-eight hours—but that's only because they were in school most of the time. They also played video games on a television for almost two and a half hours per week. This was the most television viewing by children ages two to eleven since 1995.

Experts estimate that one in three children in America are overweight or obese, and yet only 10 percent of schools offer daily physical education classes. That means 90 percent of America's children are probably not getting enough exercise.

Not so long ago, most children spent their formative years running, bicycling, monkey bar climbing, stickball playing—and dozens of other forms of outdoor play. Studies have shown that children are healthier and happier the more physical activity they get. After all, humans are bipedal primates designed by nature to be hunters and gatherers. Our ability to be physically fit, along with our ability to think, enabled us to survive; the development of our cerebral cortex and our physical activity made us the top hunter in the world.

Clearly, exercise is as critical to your child's well-being as nutrition in many ways. Children who exercise do better in terms of socialization, performance in school, and ability to focus. From a medical point of view, exercise can help build overall strength, bone density, and healthy joints and muscles; it can help prevent obesity, diabetes, high blood pressure, and, later in life, cardiovascular disease. It can also help prevent depression and anxiety. And if you're looking for a way to help relieve stress and make it easier to sleep at night, exercise is a terrific place to start.

Another important benefit of exercise that doesn't always spring to mind is that it can improve your child's psychological well-being, including gaining more self-confidence and higher self-esteem. Exercise also has positive effects on mental functions. Studies on mice have shown that those who were aerobically active showed dramatic brain growth, specifically in the hippocampus, an area in the brain associated with learning and memory. And other experiments (actually performed on children as opposed to rodents) have shown that forty minutes of aerobic exercise per day improved executive function, the aspect of intelligence that helps us pay attention, plan, and resist distractions.

When we talk about exercise for children, we are talking about being active. Adults usually picture hours in the gym, on the treadmill, or running long distances. Children often just enjoy running around. Watch children on a playground and all you see is little bodies in motion. Unless it's the absolute only last-resort option, we never recommend that children use the treadmill or other gym equipment for exercise. We'd much rather they get outdoors and just play, go bike riding or skateboarding, or join organized sports.

### How Much Exercise Do Your Children Need?

Sedentary behavior, and specifically television viewing as noted above, has in many cases replaced time children used to spend in physical activities.

It has also contributed to increased calorie consumption through excessive snacking and eating meals in front of the television.

### An Excellent Resource

Visit the National Institutes of Health's WeCan (Ways to Enhance Children's Activity and Nutrition) Web site at www.wecan.org for ideas on increasing physical activity, decreasing screen time, and improving food choices among children.

As long as there are no safety issues involved, children should have as much physical activity as possible. The National Association for Sport and Physical Education (NASPE) offers expanded activity guidelines for infants, toddlers, and preschoolers:

| Age | Minimum Daily Activity | Comments |
| --- | --- | --- |
| Infant | No specific requirements | Physical activity should encourage motor development. Dance around with your baby. Get down on the floor and play with her, encouraging her to move her arms and legs. |
| Toddler | 1½ hours | 30 minutes planned physical activity *and* 60 minutes unstructured physical activity (free play). Recommended activities include running, throwing, tag, and leap frog. |
| Preschooler | 2 hours | 60 minutes planned physical activity *and* 60 minutes unstructured physical activity (free play). Work on developing balance and hand/eye coordination. They may learn to swim or to ride a bike, and begin to participate in small-scale organized sports like T-ball. |

| Age | Minimum Daily Activity | Comments |
|---|---|---|
| Ages 5 to 12 | 1 hour or more | Break up into bouts of 15 minutes or more. Greater participation in organized sports, a few times a week. Other possibilities: enrolling in classes such as yoga, gymnastics, rock wall climbing, etc. |
| Ages 13 to 18 | 1 hour or more | More organized sports if the child desires. Group activities with friends are good at this age, such as ice skating or bowling. |

The American Academy of Pediatrics recommends that playtime for children under the age of five should include lots of running and jumping and climbing and hopping. After they start kindergarten, their cognitive and motor development can begin to handle not only the skills of organized sports but also the rules and instruction that come with it. And be sure they see it as fun, not a chore. Team sports can also be a way for kids to learn social interaction skills and build self-esteem, but be sure to pick the activity with that in mind. Team sports can be daunting and debilitating if the coach is not sensitive to developmental needs or if the kids on the team are not friendly and supportive.

Physical activity doesn't have to be sports related. Walking is the best exercise there is. A great way to get kids up and out is to give them a pedometer and teach them to count their steps. You can make it a competition with you and/or your spouse, or with the whole class at school.

**A great way to get kids up and out is to give them a pedometer and teach them to count their steps. You can make it competition with you and/or your spouse, or with the whole class at school.**

Remember that kids are not little adults and don't have the same attention span. An adult might not have any problem going on a thirty- or sixty-minute bike ride for exercise. A child might not be able to sustain the ride, either physically or mentally, for the full half hour or hour. You can always break up the ride into smaller segments of ten or fifteen minutes each.

### Be Your Kid's Fitness Guru

How do we get our kids to exercise with glee? By participating in the exercise and by role modeling. Over 90 percent of children who exercise regularly have parents that exercise regularly *and don't complain about it.* Nothing is less encouraging than hearing your parents say, "Oh boy. I guess I have to get on the darn treadmill again. Ugh!" Exercise should be fun, a thing to look forward to, a part of life like brushing your teeth and eating.

This does not mean that you need to train for a triathlon. There are many ways to get more active without compromising your busy day or your wallet. Here are a few suggestions:

- Walk everywhere you can

- Bike to the places that would take too long to walk to

- Garden if that is an option

- Play outdoor games with your kids like Frisbee, basketball, and soccer instead of Nintendo

- Jump rope

- Dance to *your kid's* favorite CD

- Organize family relay races for a prize

- Play Capture the Flag or Hide and Seek outside where running to the target is key

- Choose active family vacations rather than sedentary ones

The best advice of all? Make exercise fun. Let your children decide what kind of exercise or physical activity they want to do. The best activity is the one that you will do (that goes for both you and your kids). Don't choose a sport for your child just because it's something you love. Your child may have something totally different in mind. Whatever it takes to get him moving is a good idea.

Remember to exercise or be active with a smile on your face. If the kids see you enjoying exercise as a part of your wellness plan, it will become a lifelong part of theirs.

# Questions to Ask Your Child's Doctor

- Does it seem to you that my child manifests symptoms of stress?

- Does my child seem anxious or depressed?

- Does my child seem to have normal social interaction?

- Does my child manifest any symptoms of attentional issues (e.g., ADD or ADHD)?

- Do you have any concerns about the number of hours of sleep my child gets?

- Are there any exercise classes in the area that are geared toward and safe for my child's age?

# Chapter 14 Take-Home Points

- Wellness is a state of being that focuses on balance and health rather than disease and treatment; it means practicing all the things that keep one well, including good nutrition, exercise, stress control, and sleep management.

- Stress can have direct physical consequences on your child's body. It can cause high heart rates, sweaty palms, rapid breathing, crankiness, impatience, and vulnerability to injury and illness. Both children and adults under stress are much more prone to both acute and chronic illnesses.

- Stress for children can come from many different sources: at home, at school, with their friends and peers. This is especially true if there have been any big changes in the child's life, such as parents' divorcing, moving to a new town, or a friend or family member's being ill or dying.

- Your child may be under stress if he or she becomes whiny, clingy, and/or fearful, develops insomnia, becomes withdrawn and quiet and rarely laughs, displays a sudden onset of stuttering, is easily upset by any change in schedule or routine, develops recurring headaches, or has a chronic cough or stomach pains that usually go away on weekends.

- Children often copy what they see going on around them and pick up the unhealthy vibrations they feel from their parents and caregivers. It may be that you need to learn to deal with your stress before you can help your child learn to deal with hers.

- To help your child deal with stress, teach him what stress means and give him the vocabulary with which to express it. Help your child control her world. Set up private time with each child in your household so they feel special and know they will have a chance to confide in you. Don't necessarily try to solve their problems; just be there to listen. Set up a routine for them to follow; children like to know what to expect. Teach them simple stress relievers and don't minimize their concerns, no matter how trivial they may seem.

- Studies have shown that children get about an hour less sleep each night than they did thirty years ago. Because much of a child's brain development happens when he or she is asleep, this lost hour has an exponential impact. Sleep deprivation can lead to attention and behavioral issues in children, and it can affect their memories and their emotional well-being. Plus, children who sleep less are more likely to be overweight than children who sleep more.

- The amount of sleep your child needs depends on his or her age and individual needs.

- Exercise plays a significant role in both your child's physical health and mental well-being. Aside from building overall strength, exercise can also help prevent depression and anxiety, and can improve your child's psychological well-being, including gaining more self-confidence and higher self-esteem. Exercise also has positive effects on mental functions.

- Make exercise fun. Let your children decide what kind of exercise or physical activity they want to do. The best activity is the one that you and your child will actually do.

The next, and final, chapter focuses on ways to help you plan for your children's healthy future. We know it's not always possible to make a plan and stick to it, but this will help lay the groundwork for figuring out what to buy at the grocery store and what meals to make for your family in the week ahead.

## CHAPTER 15

# Wrapping Up the Issues: Planning for a Healthy Future

Throughout this book, we have tried to provide easy, practical answers to common nutritional dilemmas that parents frequently face, and to help you to understand that the source of many of your children's illnesses and behavioral problems may be clarified through the resources of integrative pediatrics and nutritional balance. As stated earlier, our goal is to help you and your children have a healthy relationship to food and to eating—one that is not based on tricks or fads, but is instead practical, realistic, and will last a lifetime.

We did not try to create rules for you to blindly follow; instead we offered new ways of thinking about what you eat. You learned about the properties of food, how they work in conjunction with human biology, and how they can cause a lot of distress in some cases. You discovered how to make choices for your children at home, when they're at school, and when they're out with their friends at playdates and parties.

We also have urged you, and want to reiterate now, never to make major changes all at once. It's the little things you do, one baby step at a time, that get you to your goal. That's why, in this last chapter, we're giving you a few more hints about how to put the *Food Cure* into practice. Use what is most helpful to you right now and come back to what you can do at a later time. Keep in mind that there's no such thing as a perfect parent; in fact, as *Nickelodeon's* Nick Jr. says, we are all "imperfectly perfect parents." There is definitely not an absolute right way to parent, though we are all led to believe there is. The goal is to do what's best for you and your family in the long run. But, as we've stressed throughout this book, you are the grown-up here, and you have the opportunity to make some difficult but simple choices that can help your children be their most productive, happiest, and healthiest selves.

## PLAN FOR HEALTH

Sometimes it seems that our days as parents are so busy that the task of putting together healthy meals for our family is too daunting to even consider. The problem is not so much deciding what to serve—because you usually know what's best—it's wondering what your kid will actually eat: Broccoli? No. Carrots? Maybe. Macaroni and cheese? Definitely.

Have you ever found yourself asking, "What did I feed these people yesterday? How come we're having the same meal three nights in row? Why is my refrigerator full yet I still don't have anything to feed my family?" If so, you will certainly appreciate the value of planning.

Of course, there are times when spontaneous shopping is necessary (like when you run out of an essential item), but it's usually better to have specific items in mind when you go to the market. Remember that stores are not designed to sell more fresh ingredients. They are designed to entice you into buying brightly packaged convenience foods that mean less work for you and more profit for them. These are fine for an occasional treat, but not as a steady diet (they're usually high in the three things we least want: calories, fat, and sodium). Planning helps you control what your child eats because you have a better handle on what you have at home—you can't feed your child healthy snacks if you don't have any in the fridge or pantry. Planning makes it easier to fit healthier eating into your kid's busy days (and yours, too). It also helps you:

- shop for the upcoming week

- ensure that you are providing a variety of food choices

- avoid repetition of meals and snacks

- save time by being able to prepare some items in advance

The best way to start is to make an ideal meal plan for the week ahead, remembering that life is full of last-minute changes. Remember, too, that when in doubt, try to resist the urge to order in and instead just get creative with leftovers!

Here are some tips that can make meal-planning easier:

- Before you start, look through your refrigerator and see what ingredients you already have. You'll often find that you have enough to make a pasta sauce or to add to a chili or casserole dish, which will already give you one or two meals for the week without having to shop for additional ingredients.

- Try to make at least one stew or chili-style dish that you can serve for dinner twice in a week (or for a dinner and a lunch).

- Keep a file or a notebook of dishes that your family particularly likes. That way, you can repeat meals that will keep them satisfied as well as healthy.

- Practice the old tried-and-true method of collecting recipes from friends and family as well as cookbooks and magazines. And don't forget the Internet. Whenever you have a few minutes, search for easy healthy recipes and try something new at least once a week. You'll never know what your family likes if you don't get them to try new foods.

- Try to keep your weekly plan balanced: Include one or two vegetarian meals, one meal of red meat, one or two meals with poultry, and two meals that include fish.

- Emphasize fruits and vegetables. Add bulk to your meals by including a salad at lunch and dinner if possible. Use nuts and seeds and make your own low-fat dressings to add taste and nutrition.

- Get in as much variety as possible. Keep your meals colorful— include a wide range of fruits and vegetables that are green, red, purple, yellow, and orange.

- Don't be too much of a meal plan stickler. If your plans change and you suddenly decide to go out to eat, or you're invited to a friend's house for a meal, it's no big deal. If you get home late from work and you want to order in pizza, go ahead. Just don't do it every night. The plan is there to make your life easier, not to add stress if you think you have to adhere to it exactly.

## *Sample Meal Planner*

As you will see in the sample meal planner below, each day includes three meals and two snacks. This is a guide for planning your own meals and snacks; the idea is to adapt it to suit your family's personal food preferences.

| MEAL | MONDAY | TUESDAY | WEDNESDAY | THURSDAY | FRIDAY | SATURDAY | SUNDAY |
|---|---|---|---|---|---|---|---|
| **Breakfast** | French toast made with gluten-free bread Plain or vanilla yogurt with fresh fruit slices | Oatmeal with raisins and honey Almond milk | Cold whole grain cereal with yogurt and banana slices | 2-egg omelet with one whole egg and one egg white 1/8 cup shredded cheddar cheese, 1/2 tsp. olive oil Sliced pear | ½ English muffin with peanut butter Apple slices | Pancakes with fresh or frozen berries Almond or rice milk | Cold whole grain cereal with yogurt and berries |
| **Snack** | Slices of hard cheese Sliced apple or pear | Yogurt with banana slices and sunflower seeds | Celery sticks with peanut or almond butter 8 oz. flavored rice milk | Smoothie made with 1 mashed banana and 8 oz. of rice or almond milk | Slices of hard cheese Sliced apple or pear | Organic applesauce | Smoothie made with crushed berries and 8 oz. of rice or almond milk |
| **Lunch** | Chicken salad made with chopped chicken, diced celery, and light mayo; lettuce and tomato Fresh plums | Egg salad Raw vegetable slices with ranch salad dressing dip | Vegetable soup Hummus on pita bread triangles Cucumber and carrot slices | Grilled chicken sandwich (grilled chicken on gluten-free bread with honey-mustard dressing Fresh fruit slices | Lean beef or turkey hamburger with lettuce and tomato 1/2 baked potato with small dollop of sour cream | Quinoa with roasted vegetables Lettuce, tomato, and cucumber salad with olive oil and vinegar dressing | Cheese and vegetable pizza Fresh fruit |
| **Snack** | Carrot sticks with yogurt dill dressing | Popcorn drizzled with olive oil and a touch of salt | Fresh grapes | Cucumber sticks with salsa dipping sauce | Melon wedges with plain or vanilla yogurt | Pear slices with peanut butter | Carrot and cucumber sticks with yogurt dill dressing |
| **Dinner** | Chili made with ground turkey or chicken Green salad with olive oil and vinegar dressing | Flounder sautéed in olive oil Baked sweet potato with small pat of butter or healthy spread Frozen peas and carrots | Baked chicken Steamed fresh vegetables drizzled with olive oil Quinoa Glass of water or flavored seltzer | Gluten-free pasta with roasted veggies in tomato sauce Green salad with olive oil and vinegar dressing | Baked salmon with fresh green beans Quinoa Green salad with olive oil and vinegar dressing | Turkey tacos, hard or soft (ground turkey, cheddar cheese, salsa, romaine lettuce, tomato, avocado) | Chinese stir-fry (skinless chicken breast, fresh chopped vegetables stir-fried in olive oil and light soy sauce) Steamed brown rice |

Here is a blank meal planner for you to copy and use. Put it on your refrigerator or bulletin board to keep track of the meals you plan to serve each week.

## Week of _____

| MEAL | MONDAY | TUESDAY | WEDNESDAY | THURSDAY | FRIDAY | SATURDAY | SUNDAY |
|------|--------|---------|-----------|----------|--------|----------|--------|
| Breakfast | | | | | | | |
| Snack | | | | | | | |
| Lunch | | | | | | | |
| Snack | | | | | | | |
| Dinner | | | | | | | |

Tips for menu planning:

- Include a variety of foods each day.

- Include food choices that your children will enjoy.

- For children ages two to three, include four servings per day of fruits and vegetables and three servings per day of grain products.

- For children over four years of age, include five servings a day of fruit and vegetables and four servings a day of grain products.

- Include a protein at every meal.

- Limit foods and beverages that are high in calories, fat, sugar, or salt.

- Keep serving sizes in mind. Don't serve huge portions; let your child ask for seconds of foods they enjoy.

### Guidelines

Here are some tips on how to make sure you feed your children balanced meals:

- Fill one half of your child's plate with protein (e.g., chicken, eggs, beans, lean cuts of pork or beef).

- Fill one quarter of the plate with a complex carbohydrate (e.g., brown rice, sweet potato, quinoa, couscous).

- Fill one quarter of the plate with vegetables (e.g., carrots, broccoli, cauliflower, green beans).

Here are some guidelines for serving sizes:

**Proteins:**
- 2½ oz. cooked meat, fish, or poultry

- 2 eggs

- ¾ cup cooked beans, lentils, or hummus

- 2 tbsp. peanut butter

**Grain products:**
- 1 slice bread

- 2 oz. cold cereal

- ¾ cup hot cereal

- ½ cup pasta, rice, quinoa, or couscous

- ½ bagel, pita, tortilla, or bun

**Fruits and vegetables:**
- 1 medium-size fruit or veggie

- ½ cup fresh, frozen, or canned fruit or veggie

- 1 cup green salad

**Milk and milk alternatives:**
- 1 cup cow's milk, almond milk, or rice milk

- ¾ cup yogurt

Planning menus for the week is a wonderful thing. But in real life, it may not be so easy to do. If it's too time-consuming for you, or if you're just not the organized type, don't fret. Instead, just plan to have really basic healthy food in the house as best you can and stock up (really stock up) on dried goods like quinoa as a great way to have a last-minute stir-fry with leftovers.

## ONE FINAL NOTE

It is our hope and belief that by following the *Food Cure* suggestions, your child is no longer subject to the earaches, tummy aches, fatigue, irritability, and I-don't-want-to-go-to-school syndrome that was so worrisome before you read this book. You can test it out for yourself. Once you've begun making even just a few of the simple changes laid out for you in this book, go back to Chapter 1 and take the quiz called "Is This Your Child?" You will be amazed to find that your answers to many of the quiz's questions will have already changed for the better.

# Appendix A: Resource Guide

**To contact Natalie Geary, MD:**

Integrative Pediatrician at Private Pediatric Consulting LLC

212-628-5117

vedababy@gmail.com

www.vedapure.com

www.modernmums.com

**To contact Oz Garcia, PhD:**

Oz Garcia

10 West 74th Street, Apartment 1G

New York, NY 10024

212-362-5569

info@ozgarcia.com

www.ozgarcia.com

**For information on the Bodies exhibition worldwide:**

www.bodiestheexhibition.com

**Organizations**

Food Allergy and Anaphylaxis Network

11781 Lee Jackson Highway, Suite 160

Fairfax, VA 22033

800-929-4040

faan@foodallergy.org

www.foodallergy.org

Center for Food Allergies
1229 Madison Street, Suite 1220
Seattle, WA 98104
888-546-6283
info@centerforfoodallergies.com
www.centerforfoodallergies.com

National Institutes of Health's WeCan
(Ways to Enhance Children's Activity and Nutrition)
www.wecan.org

NHLBI Health Information Center
Attention: Web site
P.O. Box 30105
Bethesda, MD 20824-0105
301-592-8573
nhlbiinfo@nhlbi.nih.gov
www.nhlbi.nih.gov

## PRODUCTS

You can find many of the products mentioned in this book in your local supermarkets and/or health food stores. If you can't find them there, try these Web sites:

### Sites for gluten-free breads and pastas:
www.glutenfreemall.com
www.glutenfree.com
www.snackwarehouse.com

### Sites for goat's milk:
www.redwoodhill.com (goat cheese and yogurt)
www.meyenberg.com (goat's milk and milk products)

**Sites for rice milk:**
www.tastethedream.com (Rice Dream products)
www.goodkarmafoods.com (rice milk and milk products)

**Sites for probiotics:**
www.biogaia.com
www.culturelle.com
www.natren.com

**Sites for organic yogurts and cottage cheese:**
www.stonyfield.com
www.stonyfield.com/yobaby
www.stonyfield.com/yobaby/yokid
www.wallabyyogurt.com
http://fageusa.com
www.horizondairy.com

**Sites for nutraceuticals for children:**
Amalaki vitamin C: www.morphemeremedies.com
Carlson for Kids Chewable Vitamin C: www.carlsonlabs.com
Cold-EEZE: www.coldeeze.com
Life Extension Zinc Lozenges: www.lef.org/vitamins-supplements
Eden Organic Seaweed Gomasio: www.edenfoods.com
Dr. Ron's Ultra Pure Blue Ice Fermented Cod Liver Oil: www
    .drrons.com
Dr. Fuhrman's DHA Purity: www.drfuhrman.com
Carlson for Kids Chewable DHA: www.carlsonlabs.com
Neuromins DHA: www.vitabase.com
Enfamil Fer-In-Sol Iron Supplement Drops (for infants and
    toddlers): www.enfamil.com
Lactoferrin Gold 1.8: www.nikken.com
NutriCology Laktoferrin: www.nutricology.com

Childlife Essentials Vitamin D3 Mixed Berry Flavor: www.vitacost
.com
Carlson Labs Baby D Drops: www.carlsonlabs.com
Thorne Research Children's Basic Nutrients: www.thorne.com
Dr. Sears Little Champions Children's Multivitamins: www
.drsearsfamilyapproved.com

**CDC site for measuring children's BMI:**
http://apps.nccd.cdc.gov/dnpabmi/

# Appendix B: Glossary

**Adaptive immunity:** This type of immunity involves lymphocytes, white blood cells that allow the body to recognize previous invaders and help destroy them. This is how vaccination works. Particular antigens (any foreign substance, such as a bacterium or virus, that stimulates an immune response in the body) are introduced to the body in small amounts. This signals the body to make antibodies (infection-fighting protein molecules) that are designed specifically to fight any future invasions of that particular antigen.

**Allergy:** An allergy occurs when your immune system reacts to a foreign substance as if it was a threat to your well-being and therefore generates antibodies. An allergy is measurable via a blood test. You may outgrow an allergy, but at the time you are allergic, eating less of a particular food won't make you less allergic to it.

**Amino acids:** Amino acids are small molecules that link together in long chains to form proteins. The proteins you eat are broken down by the digestive system into amino acids. Those amino acids are subsequently used by the body to maintain and repair tissues, blood, and bone.

**Anaphylaxis:** A sudden, severe, potentially life-threatening allergic reaction.

**Antibiotics:** A class of medications used to treat bacterial infections. Antibiotics are not effective against viral infections.

**Antibodies:** Proteins found in blood or other bodily fluids, used by the immune system primarily to identify and neutralize bacteria and viruses.

**Antihistamines:** A class of medications used to block the action of histamines (inflammatory substances produced by the body that are responsible for causing allergy symptoms) and help to minimize the symptoms of an allergic reaction.

**Antioxidant:** A substance that prevents or slows down oxygen decomposition of a material. These substances, which can come from healthy foods, protect us from many disease-causing agents.

**Atopic triad:** The atopic triad is a combination of skin, gastrointestinal, and respiratory hypersensitivities. Atopic individuals have a genetic tendency toward hypersensitive reactions to certain triggers, which can be anything your body recognizes as "foreign." This hypersensitivity usually manifests in the form of rhinitis (a non-infectious runny nose), asthma, and/or atopic dermatitis (itchy flaking patches of sensitive skin), although how much or how little of each of these three conditions a person develops tends to vary.

**Celiac disease:** People who are truly allergic to wheat may have celiac disease, a digestive disorder that interferes with the absorption of nutrients from food. Some common symptoms of celiac disease are diarrhea, decreased appetite, stomachache and bloating, poor growth, and weight loss. This is a serious disease that requires strict adherence to a gluten-free diet.

**Cytokines:** Small proteins released by cells that, among other things, help fight off infections.

**DHA:** An omega-3 fatty acid incorporated into neural and eye tissue, docosahexaenoic acid (DHA) is critical for the development and function of the brain, nerve cells, and the eyes. DHA is also important in the function and maintenance of the immune system, hormone regulation, and general health.

**Essential fatty acid (EFA):** A building block of the body necessary for human health. The body cannot make EFAs, so we must get them from the foods we eat (e.g., salmon, sardines, avocados). EFAs are critical for proper growth in children, especially for neural development and maturation of sensory systems. It's also vital that expectant mothers get adequate supplies of EFAs, as they are passed on to fetuses and nursing babies.

**Gluten:** Gluten is a protein found in wheat (including durum and bulgar) and other grains including oats, rye, barley, millet, kamut, and spelt. It binds the dough in baking and prevents crumbling. Gluten can be found in foods like breads, cakes, pastries, cookies, biscuits, crackers, battered foods, cereals, snack foods, pastas, and pizza.

**Glycemic index (GI):** A scientifically developed way to identify which carbohydrates are good for you and which are not so good. The glycemic index was designed to measure how rapidly a carbohydrate is absorbed into your bloodstream and its potential impact on insulin secretion. Each carbohydrate is assigned a number that reflects the rate at which it causes glucose (sugar) levels in the blood to rise. The higher the number, the faster the carb converts to glucose in the blood. The goal is to keep that number low.

**High-fructose corn syrup (HFCS):** Regular corn syrup that has been treated with an enzyme that converts glucose into fructose (which is sweeter). Many beverages and other processed foods made with high-fructose corn syrup and other sweeteners are high in calories and low in nutritional value.

**Homeopathy:** A system of medicine that uses highly diluted doses from the plant, mineral, and animal kingdoms to stimulate natural defenses in the body.

**Immunoglobulin E (IgE):** True allergic reactions cause the body's immune system to develop antibodies against what it perceives to be a foreign invader. This "invader" is usually a protein. The first time you ingest this protein, the immune system responds by creating specific antibodies called immunoglobulin E, or IgE. Although antibodies are usually protective, IgE antibodies can cause a broad variety of inflammatory reactions, including rash, diarrhea, stomach pains, watery eyes, etc. These reactions can range anywhere from mild to extreme; in the worst cases, allergies can be deadly.

**Inflammatory response:** A response of body tissues to injury or irritation, characterized externally by pain, swelling, redness, and/or heat. Internally, inflammation can cause the production of destructive antibodies reacting to the body and/or mucus. This is the body's normal response to abnormal stimulation caused by disease or illness. Most of us are somewhat inflamed almost all the time.

**Innate immunity:** This is immunity that we are born with. It includes the natural barriers we have to protect ourselves, like the skin and the mucous membranes that line the nose, throat, and gastrointestinal tract, which are our first line of defense against invaders.

**Integrative medicine:** Integrative medicine takes into account both Western and alternative practices, using the Eastern philosophy of looking at the whole body and wellness while still utilizing modern Western medical practices when they are indicated. Integrative medicine implies that the practitioner is trained to interpret and utilize whatever modality is best for a particular situation.

**Intolerance:** Intolerance is your body's inability to process the level of a particular food that you're asking your body to digest. An intolerance, or sensitivity, is not measurable, as antibodies are not produced. However, your body is not clearing the particular food out of your system very well. An intolerance is controllable, meaning if you eat less of a particular food to which you have a sensitivity, the body is better able to handle it and you will feel better.

**Lactose intolerance:** Lactose intolerance is a deficiency in the enzyme (lactase) that is made in your intestinal tract and is required to break down lactose (milk sugar) that you ingest. If you are deficient in this enzyme, your intestinal tract struggles to break down and process the milk sugars. This condition is not dangerous, just unpleasant, and most people, even children, will learn to avoid the foods that cause the discomfort—the bloating, the cramping, the reactive diarrhea. For these children, their body is intolerant to milk, but not allergic.

**Lectin:** Lectin is a tiny molecule that selectively causes blood and other body tissues to stick together. All foods contain lectins, but while they are benign in some foods, they are toxic in others. Foods with high concentrations of lectins, such as beans, cereal grains, seeds, and nuts, may be harmful if consumed in excess. In some foods (particularly wheat, dairy—especially when cows have been grain-fed—and legumes), lectins are more likely to cause sensitivities and/or allergies.

**Legumes:** Edible seeds or pods such as beans, lentils, and peas.

**Metabolic syndrome:** Metabolic syndrome is a cluster of conditions that occur together. You (or your child) may be diagnosed with metabolic syndrome if you have at least three of the following conditions:

- High blood pressure
- Insulin resistance
- Abdominal obesity
- High blood sugar
- Low HDL (good) cholesterol

- High triglycerides (fats in the blood)

- Inflammatory reactions in the blood

**Nufood:** Nufoods are man-made convenience foods that do not fulfill food's primary functions of providing the mortar for building healthy bodies and brains, and the nutrients we need to live longer and to live well. It's also devoid of most of the nutritional properties that have a broad range of functions in keeping us healthy.

**Nutraceuticals:** Nutritional supplements that have been shown to have pharmaceutical properties.

**Omega-3 fatty acid:** Omega-3 is a polyunsaturated EFA found in a variety of foods, including fatty fish, flaxseed oil or ground flaxseed, canola oil, walnut oil, and omega-3 fortified eggs.

**Omega-6 fatty acid:** A polyunsaturated EFA found in green leafy vegetables and in flaxseed, safflower, borage, and evening primrose oils, omega-6 stimulates fat-burning tissue in the body, encouraging calories to be burned for energy instead of being stored as fat.

**Passive immunity:** Passive immunity is temporary immunity that comes from an outside source and lasts a short time. For example, all babies have antibodies from their mothers, which give them short-term protection from diseases to which their mothers have been exposed.

**Phytochemicals:** Phytochemicals, also known as phytonutrients, are health-protecting compounds found in fruits, vegetables, and other plants. There are thousands of phytochemicals found in the plant world. While plants produce these chemicals to protect themselves, scientists have shown that they can also protect humans against diseases. Some of the best-known phytochemicals are lycopene in tomatoes, isoflavones in soy, and flavonoids in fruits.

**Probiotics:** Live microorganisms, which when given in adequate amounts, confer a health benefit on the host. Probiotics are living bacteria that are similar to the friendly bacteria found in the human intestinal system. They live symbiotically in the gut, meaning they form a give-and-take relationship where they help us fight off the bad guys in return for a warm place to live.

**Radioallergosorbent testing (RAST):** RAST involves measuring specific allergic antibodies in a person's blood. While skin testing can give a sense, based on the size of the reaction, of whether a person is truly allergic to a food, RAST actually measures the amount of allergic antibody to the food.

**Stem cells:** Unipotential cells that can form into many different types of cells depending on where they are injected or come in contact with cells that are around them. They are essentially able to grow into any cell in the body if they are employed early. This is an active area of research.

**Trans fatty acid:** The process of hydrogenating fat (when hydrogen has been artificially added to oils at extremely high temperatures to solidify them and give them longer shelf lives) causes it to change its molecular structure into what is called a trans fatty acid. Although many restaurants, fast food places, and food manufacturers are reducing or eliminating trans fatty acids, they can still be found in many commercially packaged goods, commercially fried food such as french fries from some fast food chains, other packaged snacks such as microwave popcorn, and in vegetable shortening and some margarine. Indeed, any packaged goods that contain "partially hydrogenated vegetable oils," "hydrogenated vegetable oils," or "shortening" most likely contain trans fat.

# Appendix C: Bibliography

CHAPTER 3

Barone, J., and J. R. Herbert et al. "Dietary Fat and Natural-Killer-Cell Activity." *American Journal of Clinical Nutrition* 50 (1989): 861–67.

Brolinson, D., et al. "Exercise and the Immune System." *Clinics in Sports Medicine* 26, no. 3 (2007): 311–19.

Sanchez, A., and J. L. Reeser et al. "Role of Sugars in Human Neutrophilic Phagocytosis." *American Journal of Clinical Nutrition* 26 (1973): 1180–84.

Sears, William, and Martha Sears. *The Family Nutrition Book: Everything You Need to Know About Feeding Your Children From Birth Through Adolescence.* New York: Little, Brown and Company, 1999.


CHAPTER 4

Branum, Amy M., and Susan L. Lukacs. "Food Allergy Among U.S. Children: Trends in Prevalence and Hospitalizations." Centers for Disease Control and Prevention, October 2008. www.kidswith foodallergies.org/resourcespre.php?id=129&title=food_allalle_prevalence_hospitalizations_US_children (accessed on July 7, 2009).

Cullotta, Karen Ann. "Researchers Put a Microscope on Food Allergies." *New York Times,* December 9, 2008. www.nytimes .com/2008/12/09/health/09allergies.html (accessed on August 8, 2009).

Luccioli, Stefano, and Marianne Ross et al. "Maternally Reported Food Allergies and Other Food-Related Health Problems in Infants: Characteristics and Associated Factors." *Pediatrics* 122 (October 2008): S105–S112.

**CHAPTER 5**

Basciano, H., et al. "Fructose, Insulin Resistance, and Metabolic Dyslipidemia." *Nutrition and Metabolism* 2, no. 1 (February 2005): 5.

Garcia, Oz. *The Healthy High Tech Body.* New York: Regan Books, 2001.

Jahren, Hope, and Rebecca A. Kraft. "Carbon and Nitrogen Stable Isotopes in Fast Food: Signatures of Corn and Confinement." *Proceedings of the National Academy of Sciences* 105, no. 46 (November 2008): 17855–60.

"Junk Food Babies: An Investigation into Foods for Babies and Young Children." Children's Food Campaign, May 2009. www .childrensfoodcampaign.net/CFC_Baby_food_report.pdf (accessed on July 15, 2009).

**CHAPTER 7**

"Does Cow's Milk Cause Diabetes?" *Time,* August 10, 1992. www .time.com/time/magazine/article/0,9171,976188,00.html (accessed on August 2, 2009).

"Early Man 'Couldn't Stomach Milk'." BBC. February 27, 2007. http://news.bbc.co.uk/2/hi/health/6397001.stm (accessed on August 3, 2009).

Ganmaa, D., et al. "Is Milk Responsible for Male Reproductive Disorders?" *Medical Hypotheses* 57, no. 4 (October 2001): 510–14.

Giovannucci, E., et al. "Calcium and Fructose Intake in Relation to Risk of Prostate Cancer. *Cancer Research* 58 (1998): 442–47.

"Goats' Milk is More Beneficial to Health than Cows' Milk, Study Suggests." *ScienceDaily,* July 31, 2007. www.sciencedaily.com/ releases/2007/07/070730100229.htm (accessed on August 18, 2009).

Jackson, Deborah. ". . . Or Just Go with the Flow?" *Times,* May 5, 2005. http://timesonline.co.uk.tol/lif_and_style/health/features/ article388488.ece (accessed on August 3, 2009).

Kagawa, Y. "Impact of Westernization on the Nutrition of Japanese: Changes in Physique, Cancer, Longevity and Centenarians." *Preventive Medicine* 7, no. 2 (June 1978): 205–17.

Lemay, Danielle G., and David J. Lynn et al. "The Bovine Lactation Genome: Insights into the Evolution of Mammalian Milk." *Genome Biology* 10, no. 4 (2009): R43.

"Longer Life for Milk Drinkers, Study Suggests." *ScienceDaily,* July 24, 2009. www.sciencedaily.com/releases/2009/09/090722083720.htm (accessed on August 2, 2009).

Oski, Frank A. "Is Bovine Milk a Health Hazard?" *Pediatrics* 75 (1985): 182–86.

Rich-Edwards, Janet W., and D. Ganmaa et al. "Milk Consumption and the Prepubertal Somatotropic Axis." *Nutrition Journal* 6 (2007): 28.

Simpson, A. B., and J. Glutting et al. "Food Allergy and Asthma Morbidity in Children." *Pediatric Pulmonology* 42, no. 6 (June 2007): 489–95.

Stang, Andreas, and Wolfgang Ahrens et al. "Adolescent Milk Fat and Galactose Consumption and Testicular Germ Cell Cancer." *Cancer Epidemiology, Biomarkers & Prevention* 15 (November 2006): 2189–95.

### CHAPTER 8

Dietz, William H., and Loraine Stern, eds. *American Academy of Pediatrics Guide to Your Child's Nutrition.* New York: Villard, 1999.

Harris, Gardiner. "Administration Issues New Rules on Egg Safety." *New York Times.* July 8, 2009.

*Institute of Medicine (IOM) Dietary Reference Intakes for Energy, Carbohydrate, Fiber, Fat, Fatty Acids, Cholesterol, Protein, and Amino Acids.* www.iom.edu/Reports/2003/Dietary-Reference-Intakes-for-Energy-Carbohydrate-Fiber-Fat-Fatty-Acids-Cholesterol-Protein-and-Amino-Acids.aspx (accessed on October 18, 2009).

Long, Cheryl, and Tabitha Alterman. "Meet Real Free-Range Eggs." *Mother Earth News,* Oct/Nov 2007. www.motherearthnews.com/ Real-Food/2007-10-01/Tests-Reveal-Healthier-Eggs.aspx (accessed on November 10, 2009).

Mangels, A. R., et al. "Position of the American Dietetic Association and Dietitians of Canada: Vegetarian Diets." *Journal of the American Dietetic Association* 103, no. 6 (2003): 748–65.

*USDA National Nutrient Database for Standard Reference, Release 2. Protein (g) Content of Selected Foods per Common Measure, Sorted by Nutrient Content.* www.nal.usda.gov/fnic/foodcomp/Data/SR21/ nutrlist/sr21w203.pdf (accessed on October 18, 2009).


**CHAPTER 9**

American Heart Association. "Omega-6 Fatty Acids: Make Them Part of Heart-Healthy Eating, New Recommendations Say." *ScienceDaily,* February 2009. www.sciencedaily.com/ releases/2009/01/090126173725.htm (accessed on September 9, 2009).

Birch, Eileen, et al. "A Randomized Controlled Trial of Early Dietary Supply of Long-Chain Polyunsaturated Fatty Acid and Mental Development in Term Infants." *Developmental Medicine & Child Neurology* 42 (March 2000): 174–81.

Garcia, Oz. *The Balance.* New York: HarperCollins, 1998.

*The Human Brain.* The Franklin Institute. www.fi.edu/learn/brain/fats. html#fatsbuild (accessed on August 31, 2009).

Kostyak, Dr. John, et al. "Relative Fat Oxidation is Higher in Children than Adults." *Nutrition Journal* 6, no. 1 (2007): 19.

McCann, J. C., and B. N. Ames et al. "Is Docosahexaenoic Acid, an Omega-3 Long-Chain Polyunsaturated Fatty Acid, Required for Development of Normal Brain Function? An Overview of Evidence from Cognitive and Behavioral Tests in Humans and Animals." *American Journal of Clinical Nutrition* 82, no. 2 (August 2005): 281–95.

Sheppard, Jane. "Children Need Fats to Be Healthy." *Healthy Child.* www.healthychild.com/child-nutrition/children-need-fats-to-be-healthy (accessed on August 29, 2009).

Trinkaus, Eric, et al. "Stable Isotope Evidence for Increasing Dietary Breadth in the European mid-Upper Paleolithic." *Proceedings of the National Academy of Sciences* 98, no. 11 (May 22, 2001): 6528–32.

Yehuda, S., and S. Rabinovtz et al. "Essential Fatty Acids Preparation (SR-3) Improves Alzheimer's Patients Quality of Life." *International Journal of Neuroscience* 87, nos. 3–4 (November 1996): 141–49.


**CHAPTER 12**

Eisenberg, Marla E., and Rachel E. Olson et al. "Correlations Between Family Meals and Psychosocial Well-Being Among Adolescents." *Archives of Pediatric Adolescent Medicine* 158 (2004): 792–96.

Gillman, Matthew W., and Sheryl L. Rifas-Shiman et al. "Family Dinner and Diet Quality Among Older Children and Adolescents." *Archives of Family Medicine* 9 (2000): 235–40.

Moore, Peter. "She's a Mom First." *Children's Health,* September 15, 2009. www.childrenshealthmag.com/parents/shes-mom-first.php (accessed on September 21, 2009).


**CHAPTER 13**

Begley, Sharon. "Born to Be Big: Early Exposure to Common Chemicals May Be Programming Kids to Be Fat." *Newsweek,* September 21, 2009. www.newsweek.com/id/215179 (accessed on October 7, 2009).

The Endocrine Society. "Childhood Obesity Increases Early Signs of Cardiovascular Disease." *ScienceDaily,* June 12, 2009. www .sciencedaily.com/releases/2009/06/09061114526.htm (accessed on September 30, 2009).

Freedman, D. S., and L. K. Khan et al. "Relationship of Childhood Overweight to Coronary Heart Disease Risk Factors in Adulthood: The Bogalusa Heart Study." *Pediatrics* 108 (2001): 712–18.

Goossens, Lien, et al. "Loss of Control over Eating in Overweight Youngsters: The Role of Anxiety, Depression and Emotional Eating." *European Eating Disorders Reviews* 17, no. 1 (January–February 2009): 68–78.

Harris, Jennifer L., and John A. Bargh. "Priming Effects of Television Food Advertising on Eating Behavior." *Health Psychology* 28, no. 4 (2009): 404–13.

Ludwig, David. "Childhood Obesity—The Shape of Things to Come." *New England Journal of Medicine* 357 (December 6, 2007): 2325–27.

"NHANES Data on the Prevalence of Overweight Among Children and Adolescents: United States, 2003–2006." CDC National Center for Health Statistics, Health E-Stat. www.cdc.gov/nchs/products/pubs/pubd/hestats/overweight/overwght_child_03.htm (accessed on November 3, 2009).

Olshansky, S. J., and D. J. Passaro et al. "A Potential Decline in Life Expectancy in the United States in the 21st Century." *New England Journal of Medicine* 352 (2005): 1138–45.

Taylor, C. Barr, and Susan Bryson et al. "The Adverse Effect of Negative Comments about Weight and Shape from Family and Siblings on Women at High Risk for Eating Disorders." *Pediatrics* 118, no. 2 (August 2006): 731–38.

Wake, Melissa, and Louise A. Baur et al. "Outcomes and Costs of Primary Care Surveillance and Intervention for Overweight or Obese Children: The LEAP 2 Randomised Controlled Trial." *British Medical Journal* 339 (2009): b3308.

Whitaker, R. C., and J. A. Wright et al. "Predicting Obesity in Young Adulthood from Childhood and Parental Obesity." *New England Journal of Medicine* 37, no. 13 (1997): 869–73.


**Chapter 14**

Cotman, C. W., and N. C. Berchtold. "Exercise: A Behavioral Intervention to Enhance Brain Health and Plasticity." *Trends in Neurosciences* 55, no. 3 (2002): 295–301.

Davis, Catherine, et al. "Effects of Aerobic Exercise on Overweight Children's Cognitive Function." *Research Quarterly for Exercise & Sport* 78, no. 5 (December 2007): 510–19.

Fallone, Gene, et al. "Experimental Reduction of Sleep Opportunities in Children: Effects on Teacher Ratings." *Sleep* 28, no. 12 (2005): 1561–67.

Hale, Lauren, et al. "Social and Demographic Predictors of Preschoolers' Bedtime Routines." *Journal of Developmental & Behavioral Pediatrics* 30, no. 5 (October 2009): 394–402.

Kolata, Gina. "How Much Exercise Do Children Need?" *New York Times,* September 15, 2008. www.nytimes.com/2008/09/15/health/healthspecial2/15exercise.html (accessed on October 21, 2009).

Luby, Joan L., and Xuemei Si et al. "Preschool Depression Homotypic Continuity and Course Over 24 Months." *Archives of General Psychiatry* 66, no. 8 (2009): 897–905.

Merryman, Ashley. "How to Get Kids to Sleep More." *New York* magazine, October 7, 2007. www.nymag.com/news/features/38979 (accessed on October 7, 2009).

Mindell, Jodi, et al. "Bedtime Routine: Impact on Sleep in Young Children and Maternal Mood." *Sleep* 32, no. 15 (May 2009): 599–606.

Nielsen Company. "A2/M2: Three Screen Report." October 26, 2009. http://en-us.nielsen.com/main/insights/nielsen_a2m2_three (accessed on October 27, 2009).

Van Couter, Eve, et al. "Impact of Sleep Debt on Metabolic and Endocrine Function." *The Lancet* 354, no. 9188 (1999): 1435–39.

Van Pragg, H., et al. "Running Enhances Neurogenesis, Learning, and Long-Term Potentiation in Mice." *Proceedings of the National Academy of Science* 96 (1999): 13427–31.

# Acknowledgments

*First and foremost I want to thank Sharyn Kolberg, who was not only patient but also maintained a sense of humor. This book would not be possible without her commitment, hard work, and flexibility. I would also like to thank Lara Asher for her invaluable support as editor and patient advisor. Thank you to Laura Yorke at the Carol Mann Agency for helping Oz and me to get this dream done and to Nancy Geary for teaching me what it takes to write a book. And thanks to Oz for being Oz.*

*—Natalie Geary*

*Thanks, as always, to my incredible brother Albert and his wonderful wife, Claudia. Thanks of course to my beautiful partner, Paulina, for her love and support throughout this project. Thanks to Lara Asher and Laura Yorke, and to Desiree Gruber and everybody at Full Picture. I am grateful to my remarkable staff, Randy Corwisk, Freddie Viera, and Tara Santiago, for all their help in allowing me the time to work on this book, and to Laura Powers for her dedication and support over all these years. I have to thank Sharyn Kolberg for her remarkable capabilities and her patience in crafting this book. And of course, thanks to the fabulous Natalie Geary for her knowledge, her enthusiasm, and her valued friendship.*

*—Oz Garcia*

# Index

# About the Authors

**Natalie Geary, MD,** has her own private pediatric practice in New York. She graduated *summa cum laude* in Medical Anthropology from Harvard University and received her medical degree from Johns Hopkins Medical Center. She completed her pediatric residency at New York University Medical Center and is on the faculty in Pediatrics at Columbia-Presbyterian Medical Center, Cornell-Weill Medical Center, Mount Sinai Medical Center, and NYU Medical Center. Dr. Geary is a Fellow, American Academy of Pediatrics, and a member of its committees on Child Abuse and Neglect, Adolescent Health, International Child Health, and Community Pediatrics. She is also a member of the Medical Society of the State of New York and the Johns Hopkins Medical and Surgical Association.

Dr. Geary is also the founder and president of vedaPURE, a company dedicated to infant and childhood nutrition, allergy, and wellness. Dr. Geary developed an organic skincare line for babies and nursing mothers and participates frequently in seminars and workshops for new mothers. She has extensive experience consulting and lecturing on food and skin sensitivities, nutrition and cleansing diets, and environmental health. She also lectures on child development, the socialization and emotional maturation of toddlers, cognitive and behavioral milestones, and maintenance of self-esteem throughout childhood. She is the mother of three daughters and lives and works in Manhattan and Palm Beach, Florida.

**Oz Garcia, PhD,** is recognized as the world's leading authority on healthy aging. As "nutritionist to the stars," Oz is the go-to nutritionist for A-List celebrities and Fortune 100 CEOs. His unique and customized approach to nutrition and anti-aging, coupled with more than thirty years of experience, has made Oz one of the most recognizable names in the industry. He has lectured all over the world and has been a pioneer in the study of nutrition and anti-aging.

Oz is the bestselling author of three books, *The Balance, Look and Feel Fabulous Forever,* and *Redesigning 50: The No-Plastic-Surgery Guide to 21st-Century Age Defiance.* He was twice voted best nutritionist by *New York* magazine and is frequently called upon by some of the most respected names in medicine and the news media for his up-to-the-minute perspectives on nutrition and its role in aging and longevity. Oz has been featured in prestigious publications such as *Vogue, Elle, Travel + Leisure, W* magazine, and the *New York Times.* He has also made numerous network and cable television appearances including NBC's *Today* show, CBS's *The Early Show, Good Morning America* on ABC, *20/20, 48 Hours, The View,* and Fox News.

Oz is executive chairman of Oz Wellness, LLC and has been involved in the research and development of some of the most powerful product formulations on the market. His partnership with AriZona Beverage Company has brought AM Awake and PM Relax FastShot to market. The OZ brand is also responsible for OZ Longevity Pak, OZ Brain Enhancement Sticks, and OZ Daily Boost.

Oz lives in New York City and is engaged to Paulina Shilevsky.